THE **POWER** OF **ENERGY MEDICINE**

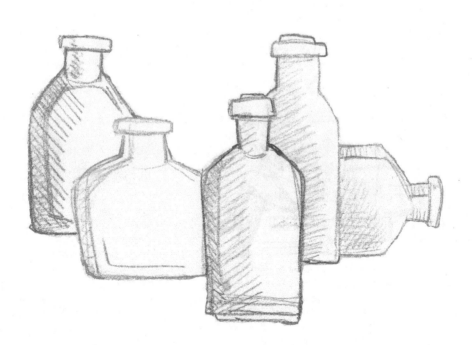

THE **POWER** OF **ENERGY MEDICINE**

Your Natural Prescription for Resilient Health

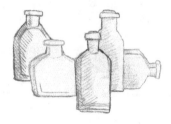

HILARY CROWLEY

Foreword by Molly Buzdon, MD

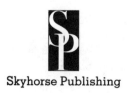

Skyhorse Publishing

Skyhorse Publishing books may be purchased in bulk at special discounts for sales promotion, corporate gifts, fund-raising, or educational purposes. Special editions can also be created to specifications. For details, contact the Special Sales Department, Skyhorse Publishing, 307 West 36th Street, 11th Floor, New York, NY 10018 or info@skyhorsepublishing.com.

Skyhorse® and Skyhorse Publishing® are registered trademarks of Skyhorse Publishing, Inc.®, a Delaware corporation.

Visit our website at www.skyhorsepublishing.com.

10 9 8 7 6 5 4 3 2

Library of Congress Cataloging-in-Publication Data is available on file.

Cover design by Daniel Brount
Cover image courtesy of Getty Images

Print ISBN: 978-1-5107-5822-3
Ebook ISBN: 978-1-5107-5938-1

Printed in the United States of America

Disclaimer: This book is a source of information only and does not constitute medical or other advice to the individual reader. This book contains the opinions and ideas of its author. Neither the author nor the publisher are liable or responsible for any injury, loss, or damage allegedly arising from this book.

Dedicated to my mom,
Judith Hunter McCann

CONTENTS

FOREWORD
by Molly Buzdon, MD

I was fortunate to meet Hilary years ago after I moved to New Hampshire in 2007. Although my formal surgical training has been in the Western tradition, I have been interested in alternative forms of medicine, and have had the good fortune to count among my friends a number of people who can view and help heal the human body in other ways than I. I was drawn to Hilary's boundless energy, enthusiasm, and powers she has to perceive that which is not physically apparent, but hiding under layers of buried traumas, fighting to stay hidden. At a young age, my son told me that he was struggling with a stressful situation that was affecting his overall well-being. When traditional therapies had not alleviated the problem, I introduced him to Hilary. She was able to navigate my son through uncharted grief in a manner that was profoundly helpful. My son shares a special bond with Hilary and still requests occasional energy "tune-ups." I myself have had a number of sessions with Hilary. I always benefit from the beautiful energy that flows out of our meetings. I often end with cleansing tears which provide a major release, leaving me more insightful, calm, and at peace.

I have always thought that the Western view of medicine leaves out too many important variables that can affect a patient's ability to heal. In my field of general surgery, the same operation can have different outcomes. I believe this can be due to different physical or mental shifts in energy. I still recall a case when I was an intern in my first year of general surgery training. An elderly gentleman was admitted with abdominal pain. He had recently lost his wife of over fifty years. An operation was being performed to investigate his abnormal CT scan finding. When my attending surgeon performed the laparotomy, looking into the abdominal cavity, cancer was seen studding all the organs. Often times, metastatic cancer can be nearly invisible on imaging studies, only apparent as small little nodules on the surface of the liver and the surrounding organs. The surgeon closed the abdomen and once the patient awoke a short time later, he gently gave the patient the diagnosis of metastatic cancer, probably arising from the stomach. I remember the patient's peaceful attitude, and when given the options of further treatment, he emphatically expressed that he did not want to pursue any further treatment. He requested a DNR, a do not resuscitate order. The next day, his lab values showed his kidneys and clotting system basically stopped working. His oxygen level dropped, indicating his lung function was declining rapidly. There was no reason for this to happen so quickly other than that he had simply decided that he did not want to live any longer. I remembered how alarmed I was at this. I wanted to try to repair all of these organ systems, but he as a single entity had already made up his mind that he did not want to live anymore. He expired the following day. My rational brain could not understand how this could happen. As physicians, we are trained to support patients and do what we can to make them better, but in the end, it is not the physician who decides if a patient lives or dies. Our most important job is determining what the patient really wants.

The entire field of medicine continues to change through leaps and bounds with advances in technology and new medications and drugs designed to cure or at least beat back cancers that have seemingly taken over the body. As we learn and discover more, I hope we also become more aware of the invisible energy that surrounds us and the part it plays in our healing and connection with ourselves and each other.

PROLOGUE

Alone in this world, each of us carried our personal medicines.

Long ago we came together, and one of us in each tribe carried the medicine. The remedies were in sacks and satchels. The memories of generations of healing wisdom existed in the heart and the mind of the medicine person.

Now, our tribes are too big to hold us together; we are alone again. This is the time to restore the memories of how we heal ourselves. Each of us has the good medicine of wisdom from our own beginnings. Our bodies hold the wisdom of our own health. We are always healing, from our starting moment to our finish line.

I've been collecting my remedies, too. The remedies were revealed as my prescription for health for myself and for the ones who work with me. I've gathered them together for you in this book.

I found medicine bottles in the doctor's bag my grandmother carried to her patients' house calls. The bottles seemed empty at first. They are full of knowing and remembering that I belong to a family who has held the medicine for the tribe.

Take what you need from these pages, refill these bottles, and reclaim your own healing. Maybe you want to carry the medicine, too.

❧

Energy medicine in health care has become more popular since I began my practice. As I prepared to explain this to a new client, Dr. Chase, a leading surgeon in the Boston area, it occurred to me that it was no longer necessary to say this is a healing art "widely received" in health care when many of my clients were medical doctors themselves. My schedule is filled by licensed therapists, health-care practitioners, and registered nurses. In fact, Dr. Chase was recommended to me through her colleague.

"Just so you know," I told Dr. Chase when we met, "I never diagnose or interfere with medical recommendations."

"Yes, I read that on your intake page," she said with no hint of resistance or even skepticism in her voice.

"Humans have written about the subtle energy fields that surround all living beings for thousands of years," I began. "Historically, human energy has been depicted in many ways—from spinning wheels of light called chakras in Sanskrit, to a cocoon of heat known as the aura. Artistic depictions of halos are inspired by the glow of heightened energy around a person's crown. The energy field exists in the lexicon of many cultures."

Dr. Chase nodded.

"When I was first introduced to energy healing, I felt entirely disoriented. No one had ever told me about this stuff as a child," I explained. "But my job involves connecting with this subtle but powerful field. When I work, my hands feel the warmth and gentle shifts right around the body, like the sensation of a magnet being pulled toward or repelled by an object. Meanwhile, my heart filters waves of joy and grief as well as impressions beyond words."

Dr. Chase listened.

"I'll try to communicate what comes through clearly—I mostly focus on the sensation in my hands. There is always useful healing information available," I said.

I invited Dr. Chase to take her shoes off to recline on the massage table in my office.

"I'm going to be moving my hands about eight inches above the surface of your body, starting at your feet, including your shins, and then your knees, your abdominal area, your neck and forehead and crown area. If you see my hands in the air, I'm balancing, clearing, receiving information . . . it's hard to describe, I'm just doing the energy work."

Then I paused, searching for the right words, but the doctor put up her hand playfully as if to say stop.

"You don't need to explain all this to me," she smiled. "I'm a surgeon. I witness this energy all the time."

"You do?" I chimed back.

"Yes. In the operating room, I always sense an undeniable presence. It's uncanny," the surgeon explained, "as if my anesthetized patient's energy is present in the room and around me while I work. It's very protective. I have no question about this energy stuff. I get it, and I believe in it. That's why I'm here."

"Good," I said, "then let's get started."

After that, I was free to do my work.

There is so much more than skin that holds me together.

—*Michael Scrogin*

chapter 1

THE HOUSE CALL

"Please say yes to the tea and cookies when you're offered," my grandmother instructed as she drove us down Spring Street. "I'll need you to wait in Mrs. Waverly's kitchen while I examine her eyes in the living room."

"But I don't drink tea," I reminded her with a smile. "Can I have chocolate milk?" Grammy, who was known in this town as Dr. Hunter, was taking me on a house call in 1978.

"Maybe they'll have some milk. You can ask. But the tea will already be waiting. I may be with Mrs. Waverly for quite a few minutes. Mr. Waverly called me early this morning. He's very concerned about her sight. She has glaucoma and is complaining about headaches. I need to rule out a few complications." She spoke in a way that made me feel grown up. I had no idea what glaucoma was, and to "rule out" sounded like an expression serious enough to stop arguing about tea.

We arrived at the Waverlys' house. I stood next to my grandmother in my green Izod shirt and red sneakers as she firmly held my left hand while carrying her doctor's bag in her other hand. Grammy was dressed up, as usual, in a tailored skirt and a silk blouse with sensible heels. She let me ring the doorbell.

Mr. and Mrs. Waverly answered the door together expectantly. My grandmother immediately walked through the room with her patient. I sat down at the kitchen table. Waiting for me was a full pot of tea, a teacup, a pitcher of cream, a bowl of sugar, and a plate of gingersnap cookies. Mr. Waverly asked me about my school vacation and mentioned how much he appreciated these doctor's visits for his wife. I thought about how this was the best way to spend

1

a vacation. I liked being out of school. I really liked seeing another world beyond my life in third grade.

"I like going to work with my Grammy," I answered.

A long time passed, and maybe it was all the caffeine and sugar, but I began to feel jittery and didn't finish the last cookie. Mr. Waverly worked at the sink as I began to wonder if "glaucoma" was even more serious than I imagined. *What did she say about complications?* I didn't hear any voices from the next room. *Where did they go?* I wanted to press my ear to the dining room door, but I thought that would be too childish.

"Could you do me a favor?" Mr. Waverly asked as he slowly brought my empty teacup to the sink. I nodded.

"Pixie is hungry, could you get her food from the breezeway?" Pixie must have known her own name because a gray cat, who I'd mistaken for a life-size figurine, pounced down from the shelf to follow me to her dish.

As I fed the cat, I forgot to watch the clock, and before I knew it the door swung open. I turned with surprise as Mrs. Waverly returned.

"Thank you, Doc," she smiled, holding the door for Grammy.

"Just keep the compressions on for an hour during the evening, for six nights," my grandmother instructed as she followed Mrs. Waverly.

I stood by the front door, eager to wave goodbye. But Mr. Waverly offered more tea and my grandmother accepted. We visited for another ten minutes before it was time for the two of us to leave for her office on Main Street.

Back in the car, my grandmother gently thanked me. "It's good to have you on these house calls. Children bring joy, you know. I like to check on my patients' health, but also, I get to check in on their whole life."

Nodding my head at nine years old, I wondered to myself, *What's the difference?*

THE GOOD MEDICINE OF GENUINE PATIENCE

Medicine Bottle #1

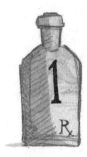

THE HOUSE CALL

When I was only nine years old, I wanted to listen through the Waverlys' door to hear my grandmother's voice. But I didn't dare try for fear it would be too childish.

But what if I had pressed my ear against the door?

What would I hear? And why did the appointment take so much time?

What would happen if *you* had plenty of time to discuss your health with your provider of care? List three topics you'd want to discuss with your doctor to check up on the whole of you.

1. _____

2. _____

3. _____

This is your prescription for the Good Medicine of Genuine Patience.

May experience a calming sensation and increased listening skills when you allow focus on your own health.

chapter 2

THE KNEE AND THE EAR

Clara and her mother arrived in my office seeking help for Clara's sleep issues and chronic knee pain. She was six years old. When I asked Clara what she thought she may need to sleep better, she quickly listed: pink bedding, a draped canopy, and a blue crystal at her bedside. We adventured into her imagination for a better night's sleep. We pretended it was bedtime. As her eyes closed and her breathing deepened, she was believably asleep, and then she giggled a little chirp, and we all laughed together. We practiced this several more times.

I asked Clara to *please* try to stay asleep at night because a good night's sleep will help her grow strong. After clearing the area of her sixth chakra which had been blocked, we gave her mom a list of ideas to transform her bed into a princess' lair. It was a light and relaxing session that vibrationally matched Clara's youthful essence.

The sixth chakra is located beneath the forehead, and it connects the mind to body consciousness. As Clara's forehead acted like a magnet pulling me to her sixth chakra, I considered this must be a particularly important chakra area for unstable sleep habits. A blocked chakra feels dense, like a humid breeze, where an unblocked chakra can feel like it's emitting energy freely, like the fresh air after a thunderstorm.

As I began to write notes to wrap up the session, Clara's mom reminded me to check in about her daughter's knee issue. I was so enveloped in the sleep issue, I was grateful for her mom's reminder. I put my hands over Clara's right knee.

Keeping the conversation light as I concentrated on the knee, I asked

Clara to talk more about sleep and describe the best dreams she could imagine. While I listened to Clara's songlike description of a princess land, I felt a buzzing warmth around her knee, a sensation I associated with molecular healing in the affected area. I paid attention and put my hand right over the kneecap.

Then something strange happened to me. My left ear began to throb. It was the inner ear, and it was distracting me. The sensation pulsed enough to cause me to shift my jaw back and forth to alleviate the pain. It subsided as I focused on the knee. Then my ear hurt again. I pulled my hands away and felt some relief. When I concentrated back to Clara's knee, my ear again began to throb.

This cycle repeated for three long minutes. Clara's mom sat across from me, watching intently as her six-year-old was relaxing with her eyes closed. Her mom must have noticed my odd twists and head tilts. I couldn't believe my ear was hurting when I only had a few more minutes left with Clara. I prepared to dismiss myself from the room to take a minute to pull and tug and massage my ear. Right at the moment I was getting ready to walk out of the room to check my ear, I remembered, *wait, this is about Clara's body communicating with me.*

It's called clairsentience. I've experienced it with other clients, too— stomachaches, headaches, joint pain, and even emotional pain. It's what I now call blueprinting—laying a picture of the client's body over my body to point out an exact area needing attention. It's always a spontaneous event. I don't intend it, and I can not conjure it. It's not a reliable technique; it just happens. That's why it surprises me, every single time, and I'm always initially confused, assuming I'm having my own physical body event.

A year earlier, I had left my office a total of *five* times during a session to remove a piece of glass that wasn't actually in my toe. A new client had booked an appointment to address her symptoms of Lyme disease, and it's noteworthy that she was still wearing shoes when I shook her hand in greeting. I kept excusing myself to the hallway to check for blood on my big toe. I was experiencing sharp pain. I was sure there was glass in my shoe. Finally, with no evidence of blood, no wound, and no glass in my toe, I considered the possibility of clairsentience.

I finally asked my client about *her* toe, and she simply replied, "It's been badly infected for a long time." In fact, it was so chronically infected, she connected it metaphysically to a deep resentment toward her previous abusive marriage. Her intuition was abundant around this toe. She opened up and began talking about her ex-husband, the abuse, and her constant pain. But I was concerned about the actual infection being addressed by a medical doctor, since I could feel it myself, and it was painful.

As soon as this new client acknowledged her own infection, my toe felt like my own again, healthy and pain-free, and we got to some productive energy healing around Lyme disease, her ex-spouse, and her toe infection. It was as if her toe was shouting, "Pay attention to me first! Please help!"

Now with Clara's ear, I had a similarly intense experience.

My left ear throbbed each time I brought my hands near Clara's knee. After my initial confusion, I cleared my mind of expectations, because I am not diagnosing—I am simply following the sensation to address the pain. I'm listening to Clara's body with my whole body.

I finally asked Clara's mom, "What's going on with Clara's ears? Especially her left ear? I'm focusing on her knee, and all I can feel is a painful sensation pulling my attention to the ear. Has she had an ear infection?"

Without pause, she replied, "Clara has had about sixteen ear infections throughout her life."

I walked toward Clara's head and hovered my hands around her ears. Perhaps her ears were saying, "Me first, me first," too.

"Does she have an ear infection now?" I wondered out loud to her mom. It was nice having a living earthly guide standing right next to me. That's really what a good parent is in the highest sense: a human guardian angel.

"Not that I know of," she answered thoughtfully.

Then my knee began to gently ache and that pulled my attention away from Clara's ears.

I went back to the knee and my ear hurt again. I repeated this until I decided to conclude that the knee issue was connected to the ear issue.

But that is about all I knew. I had no further knowledge and could offer no opinion and no hypothesis. It's not my job. My job is to connect, listen, and clear with energy healing. Clara's energy field gave me a couple strong clues to take to the chiropractor down the hallway. I felt grateful to be part of an integrative medical office where practitioners all work together. Usually we're all busy with office doors kept closed doing our work—but the nature of this working environment requires that we seek to share and help each other whenever possible. At this moment, my ear hurt and I was professionally stumped, but just because *I* couldn't interpret the connection between a throbbing ear and a sore knee, that didn't mean Clara was at a roadblock. Collaboration is vital. I would gather more resources.

As I zipped down the hall from the old building to the new wing, I hoped the doctor would see me for a quick interchange. Chiropractors are generally open to the wonders of the energy body. In fact, the chiropractors I've talked to describe good energy flow as crucial for proper alignment, which is a major factor in authentic health. The truth at that moment was that I really didn't care if our chiropractor believed me or not. I would be translating for a six-year-old girl's wisdom body as it succinctly communicated to me, "If you want to help my knee, then help my ear." I needed to try.

§

Chiropractors know ears really well. Ears require structural alignment to perform correctly. When my first son was three years old, we spent a whole night in our hospital's emergency room because he was crying and vomiting and reported that his face hurt. The ER doctor confirmed an ear infection and prescribed antibiotics. At four in the morning, I picked up the prescription, but by nine o'clock my son still couldn't ingest it with his nausea. Frankly, that was fine with me because the sun had risen, and I could take him to his primary care practitioner, whom I'll call Elisabeth.

I remain 100 percent grateful to the emergency physician from the night before. This ER doctor's calm presence and gentle approach when, in the middle of the night, I was terrified by all the possible reasons my son's whole head could be experiencing acute pain, was my life line for those hours. His professional care, his keen diagnosis, and the prescription he wrote were what we needed to get through the night. He prescribed a dropper that reduces pain—an ibuprofen drug that goes directly into the ear, which worked well to mitigate the local pain. That morning in her office, Elisabeth reminded me to put garlic oil in my son's ear to alleviate the infection. "If you can't get to a chiropractor by this afternoon, begin the antibiotics," she said firmly.

My chiropractor, Dr. Judy, lived thirty minutes away, and we had a family appointment scheduled in two days. Could this wait two days? I asked.

But Elisabeth shook her head, "You need to find a chiropractor in the next couple of *hours* for this ear infection or start the antibiotics right away. Your son has a bolus, red inflammation, in there." She had the ear scope lit and shining right into the infected ear. "And once you start the antibiotic, you need to finish the whole cycle. Don't stop just because the symptoms subside. Plus, you'll need to give him a strong probiotic, too."

As I thought about getting doses of medicine into my little child every day for two weeks, my motivation to find an available chiropractor in the area grew quickly—even in my sleep-deprived state. I called Dr. Judy. She answered her own office phone and immediately offered to help my son if I could arrive in the next hour.

My son was whimpering when we left New Hampshire and drove across the Massachusetts border, but the pain drops and garlic were helping, and soon he fell asleep. I dreaded waking his exhausted body to bring him into her office. She has a beautiful brick building hidden behind a wall of lilac bushes. I had almost succeeded in carrying his sleepy body inside when we were greeted by Dr. Judy's two fluffy, bouncy, standard poodles with barks loud enough to wake my son fully.

My son clung to my shoulders and tucked his head to my neck as I sat among the other patients in the waiting area. Right away, Dr. Judy stepped out and asked us to come in. We were the most recent patients to arrive in the full room, but the first to be seen by the doctor. I looked back apologetically at the others waiting quietly and felt a generosity of spirit from the whole group. Kindness really does help the hardest days along.

I didn't know what I expected regarding the treatment. I wondered if the chiropractor was going to adjust his neck with an undeniable crack like she did for me. Once I was face-to-face with Dr. Judy, I was delighted to discover that she was merely going to be using a pen-like compressor around my son's ear.

It happened in less than two minutes. "Click, click, click, click, click . . ."

"OK," said Dr. Judy confidently, "he should be feeling better shortly. Call me, and I'll do it again tomorrow if he's not all clear by tonight." I couldn't rationalize how a few clicks could offset the painful inflammation that had tormented him through the night.

As I quickly wrote out a check, my son walked back through the waiting room. Ten strides ahead of me now, he stopped and turned and asked, "Can you taste that, Mom?"

"No, buddy," I was chasing him as he ran to the exit, "I can't taste what you taste."

"It's dat stuff in my ear," he said in his three-year-old way.

"Oh, the garlic," I said, "How does your ear feel now?"

"All better, let's go out," he exclaimed.

I looked back at Dr. Judy with no words except a hand over my mouth to keep me from crying out with gratitude. With a waiting room of people as my witnesses, I experienced one of the fastest transformations from sickness to health I'd ever seen.

∂₹

Chiropractors know about ear infections. When I approached my colleague down the hallway, she was fortuitously available at her desk. I explained that Clara was six years old and, according to her mom, had had sixteen ear infections. I added that Clara's knee hurt to the point where she was scheduled to see a rheumatologist in Boston. I described connecting "energetically" to her knee, and how her body kept demanding to express, "the knee pain is connected to the ear pain."

"Does any of this make sense?" I asked.

Without hesitation, Dr. Kursten simply answered, "Absolutely."

I took a step back in relief and listened as she methodically hypothesized that Clara didn't have sixteen ear infections but, more likely, she explained, one lifelong ear infection that had never fully cleared. As a six-year-old, Clara's body may have adjusted off center, which could cause undue stress on that knee. Basically, the ear infection had thrown off her fundamental balance and alignment.

I rushed back down the hallway to Clara and her mom.

When I came back into my room, Clara was playing with the stones in the zen garden tray on a side table. "I was stumped," I said, "but I may have an answer for you."

"Really?" Clara's mom perked up with an inquisitive smile.

"It's possible that the ear infection has created a misalignment of Clara's body that has somehow put an undue burden on her knee." I continued to tell the whole explanation given by Dr. Kursten. I offered to introduce Clara to Dr. Kursten, and we walked down the hall together. When we arrived in her office, Dr. Kursten got down on her knees to Clara's level and explained that she was "the mommy of twin girls the same age." Clara's mom gave me a warm hopeful smile as I excused myself to get back to my office to prepare for my next client. Then I turned back, thinking twice, and gave Clara a hug.

"Thank you, Clara. You are one smart girl, and I learned a lot from you today." I smiled and we waved goodbye to each other as she held her mom's hand.

When I followed up with Clara two months later, her mom reported that her knee pain was gone and the rheumatologist gave her an all-clear prognosis. Now, years later, Clara's mom told me her daughter has not had an ear infection since that day.

THE GOOD MEDICINE OF COLLABORATION

Medicine Bottle #2

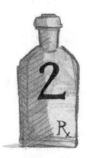

THE KNEE AND THE EAR

One powerful lesson from Clara's session involved reaching out to others for help. And another important lesson is about being available when people reach out to you for help.

When Dr. Kurston got on her knees to meet Clara eye to eye, she was intentionally connecting with her on a deeper level.

For this dose of good medicine, go out of your way to see someone eye to eye who needs your attention: a friend, a younger child, a student, a patient, a client, a customer, a pet, a loved one, a family member, or a neighbor.

How does connection enrich your abilities to help others? List three ways you can make a difference in someone else's life with your talents and abilities.

1. _____

2. _____

3. _____

This is your prescription for the Good Medicine of Collaboration.

May experience faster results and sudden urges to become active in solutions. Daily intake is appropriate.

chapter 3

VITAL SIGNS

The morning was cloudless and the bright autumn sky ignited the New Hampshire foliage. The visitor parking lot was full by seven o'clock. The hospital's educational coordinator told me to expect sixty attendants for this morning's lecture. With both hands full of materials, I briskly passed the front desk attendant and waited for the elevator. Up I went. I knew my way to the wards in this hospital: obstetric, pediatric, acute care, internal medicine. But where was the educational room located? As if by habit, I went up to the third floor, looked at the nurses' station, reconsidered my location, and went down the elevator. There was a map on the panel wall that showed my event location was to the right, just a few steps away from the front entrance. It occurred to me that I was more comfortable on the hospital floors with patient rooms than in the big meeting areas where I was expected to speak to an audience. I always looked forward to my hands-on energy work, but this morning at the hospital my job was to *describe* energy healing.

Portsmouth Regional Hospital was the first American hospital to offer energy healing in the form of Reiki. I expected my talk would be well received, but I was still outside my comfort zone describing energy healing to a large group.

By eight o'clock, the room smelled like coffee and was filled with friendly chatter that sounded like everybody was ready for a party. A nurse administrator introduced me. "Please welcome Hilary Crowley, who is here to speak about Energy Medicine and the Intelligent Healing Body," she said. The group greeted me with quiet acceptance as I noted a particular sort of curiosity settling into the room.

"Thank you for including me here at this hospital. I've always felt at home in hospitals," I began. "This morning, I get to speak on a topic I'm passionate about in this setting, where I've actually been both a patient and a caregiver.

"I love my work, and I'm grateful to talk about being an energy worker in an integrative setting. I want to start by answering this question: What in the world is energy work in an integrative setting?"

A few people in the audience gave encouraging shrugs as I continued.

"These ancient practices of the laying on of hands, studying energy centers, mapping paths in the body, and connecting the physical to the nonphysical, have emerged to a level of popularity that has raised a collective curiosity in health care.

"But why *has* it become popular? In my experience, the answer is simple: because often when energy healing is involved, patients report to feel better. Feeling better matters. Energy medicine, in all forms, remains on the margins of medicine, and maybe that's the best place for it to dwell. Starting with the glaring omission from the health insurance payment system, energy medicine is not fully validated." I kept talking as the audience sipped more coffee.

"Being in the proverbial 'alternative' role," I continued, including the air-quotes with my fingers, "is like sitting on the playground wall watching the popular kids play kickball. We may be asked to play, we may not. But we are present for the game. Even just to watch until we have access to the field. In this corner of health care, my clients tend to be open-minded, yet skeptical. It's an important word. Not cynical, but skeptical. Cynical is defined as 'distrustful of human sincerity and integrity.' Skeptical means 'not easily convinced, having doubts, or reservations.' I value skepticism.

"We *need* to care about the outcome and not be easily convinced. I'm only here in my career to assist each and every client in their own healing abilities.

"Recently, I found a popular article about the 'highly debunked' theory of life force energy as a medicine to cure disease and illness. The more I searched for scientific context for life force, the less researched substance I found. I was discouraged on behalf of the patients and medical professionals that may be asking the same questions and seeing these same sources.

"Nevertheless, even without enough present scientific data yet to show, this is my passion, and I push through my own skepticism because the benefits are profound—I teach about how utterly valid this question 'does the body's energy force matter?' actually is. I've been a student of this question my whole life. I look forward to this work someday being validated in the medical community. But for my purposes, it's just been a matter of helping one person at a time.

"Then, recently, at the most extraordinary moment, I got an answer—it happened right at Boston's very own Massachusetts General Hospital."

I paused for a moment as I began to recall the moment.

"It wasn't the answer I was expecting . . . ," I said.

We all shared our first nervous laugh together. All of us seemed not exactly sure what the other was laughing about.

"My mother was dying." I shifted into the story. "After three intense months of failing health, she was at Harvard University's big teaching hospital. And here was my mother at this great hospital. Her dignity, her comfort, and ultimately, her peaceful death was my primary concern. Over those last months, I slept by her side at three different hospitals and stayed with her when she was home. My sister and I never left her unattended for the entire time, even when she was under the watchful eye of private nurses and the care of my dad.

"In her last week of life, she was sent back to Massachusetts General Hospital. The monitors were off, she was heavily medicated, and in a semi-coma state. No longer speaking and no longer needing any moment-to-moment caregiving from me because now not only was my dad ever present but also, my two brothers had arrived and watched over her in vigil. And even still, my sister stayed by her side.

"I was with my mother knowing it was the last time I'd see her and it was almost time for me to leave and return home to my children. I pulled the attending doctor aside and asked him, 'How does this work now? How does she die? Is her liver failing? Last week we thought the tumor on her skull may be putting pressure on her brain. When does the brain stop sending signals? Is it renal failure? What is going to actually cause her death?'

"The doctor was tall and looked really young to me. His body language showed that he was in a respectful hurry. He turned to make eye contact and answered, 'we actually don't know; only the body knows. The human body knows exactly how to die. Notice how we turned her monitors off. . . . There is nothing to do now. She seems peaceful, and we don't know what steps her body is taking right now. The body is wise,' he said sagely, 'and you can trust that. There is nothing else to monitor. There is powerful energy at work here. Her body knows how to *do its thing*. She is in good hands.'

"I looked down," I told my audience, "and an inexplicable lightness came over me. I took a breath and simply said 'thank you' as I watched his white coat rush away to his next patient. With a view of my mother's fading body surrounded by her family, I silently promised myself to remember this moment and the validity of this energy healing work I do. What I know by engaging with the subtle energy body is that I bring healing insight, stress relief, and balance that assists the body to *'do its thing'* every day of my life.

"We are moving, breathing, feeling, thinking circuit systems," I said. "We are still mysterious. Our potential to heal is mostly untapped."

I turned away to get a sip of water, check my notes, and catch myself from breaking into tears. My mother's death was only months behind me and my grief was still raw and palpable. I knew I just needed to keep speaking to keep from crying. I turned back and continued.

"Integrative medicine is the star that I swing from. I think surgery is an absolute gift to humanity, and medicines that can augment organ function, bring pain relief, and accelerate healing are the miracles of our time in history . . ."

I looked around and suddenly felt unsure. I began again.

There was a strong energy in the room that I could not decipher. I scanned the room and asked, 'Does anyone have any questions?'"

A woman in the second row quickly raised her hand.

"Yes?" I was eager to answer her question.

She asked, "Could we take a bathroom break?"

I looked to the coordinator for permission to stop for a few minutes. She agreed it was a good time to take a five-minute break.

My mind raced. I wondered if I missed a step with my presentation. I rechecked my notes wondering if I should have prepared differently. Maybe it was just too early in the morning to be on this topic. I wanted to slip out the back door and I suspected everyone else did, too. I walked over to my colleague who was watching me from her chair while others scurried for coffee during the short break.

"This isn't going well," I said to her as the blood rushed out of my face.

"What do you mean? It's fine, it's great, just get to the good stuff," she said cheerfully.

"I don't know how to *talk* about the good stuff," I said.

"Sure you do," she gently argued. "Just keep going, you'll be fine."

But I didn't feel like it would be fine. I'm an energy worker, after all, and I could feel that the energy was not flowing quite right yet.

After the break, the seats were full again. To my sincere relief, it looked like everyone came back for the second part. And at that exact moment, I decided to change the second part.

"Thanks for allowing me that lengthy introduction, but I think I'm done lecturing." I started up again. "Now I need to go back to my roots. It's time to just show how the body heals. I'm not sure how I'm going to do this, but I'm tossing the rest of my notes to the side . . ."

I moved all my paperwork and the white board easel into the corner. In its place, I brought one single chair to the front of the room.

"I need a volunteer," I smiled, feeling my confidence return. My colleague gave me a knowing nod of encouragement.

Suddenly four, then six, and then eight hands went up. This was a good sign. I chose the volunteer right in the second row; the same person who asked for a bathroom break.

"I'm relinquishing my agenda and I'm going to let our energy bodies be the teachers. But here is my last nugget; three mindsets can always support your healing. Hope, Gratitude, and Forgiveness. You choose one of these three, and I'll ask your body's wisdom to teach all of us more about the one you chose."

"Forgiveness," the volunteer looked up at me from the chair.

I knew this would work, but at the same time I also had no idea if this would work. Confident and cautious, I really needed the energy to come through for this tough audience. I may just go blank again. I knew this. My nerves were still fairly tense with the pressure.

"I'm going to be silent for a few moments," I said to everybody, "and it may seem a bit awkward, but hang in there, and I'm going to do my work."

I scanned my hands over the volunteer's head and felt her strong energy field with a pull toward her neck area. Carefully, I floated my left hand in front of her voice box as I held my right hand behind her upper back. A picture flashed in my mind's eye of a baby stroller and a woman texting on her phone . . . as if, instead of looking at her baby or holding the baby, she was staring into the mobile phone. This image repeated in my mind like a film trailer clip. I felt a heavy emotion of grief, not around an actual death, but definitely a a significant loss. Like a magnetic force, I felt this heaviness leave from the shoulders and neck area as the energy balanced around her.

"Take a deep breath," I said quietly.

"I think I'm going to cry," she whispered back.

Suddenly, in my second difficult epiphany of the morning, I remembered how private this energy healing can be.

And so I said to everyone, "This is energy work, and I'm going to ask you to support us energetically in these next few moments. Just send good thoughts our way. Is that OK?" I felt the group lean toward us with a comforting murmur of support.

My volunteer felt the support, too, as she gently began to cry more freely. Her experience felt *exceptionally* private. "Thank you for bravely volunteering—you probably didn't expect this."

"I didn't know what to expect but," she spoke up. "I needed help with this one, this forgiveness. I think I knew this might happen."

"Well, it still feels important to keep this private, but can I share one small general insight that showed itself?"

She nodded, and I began to teach the audience *from* her body's wisdom.

"In this age of distraction, we need to look at loved ones in their eyes. Whether it's a child in a stroller or a person you're writing a message to. There is a block here that's all ready to open up and clear once you allow your eyes to connect with others. In general," I turned to the volunteer, "your body is showing us that there are important issues that aren't going to be solved by texting. I feel your body is saying, 'please less texting and more connecting.' Authentic connection is the most crucial part of all relationships. That's your message for us."

Still the guest speaker, I felt entirely out on a limb from where my presentation began, and yet I felt more confident. I was finally *showing* how energy gets down to the roots of healing. But for this to work, there had to be a piece about the forgiveness my volunteer chooses to explore. That's when I asked everyone to pay close attention to the next answer.

"Does this experience connect with forgiveness? How can we learn from you?" I asked her.

"Oh, it most definitely connects to forgiveness," she exclaimed, "most definitely."

And then she looked at everyone seated in front of her. "But this is really private," she apologized, "no one could have known about this issue, and it's about my child, so I'm sorry I can't share it in detail. But this is all very healing—what she's saying and what I'm feeling. Trust me."

The volunteer went back to her place in the audience as the room leaned back and gave her some space.

For the rest of the presentation, we went on to learn and share more about forgiveness, gratitude, and hope from five different volunteers until we ran out of time.

I closed by sharing, "Wherever you are in your life and in your health, you can always access this deep well of wisdom. Our bodies are here to serve us at all levels and at all times. Trust your body to 'do its thing,' not just at the end of life, but in all the vital moments of health and well-being along the way."

As I said goodbye, the first volunteer approached me again and asked to speak privately. "You said the word 'vital.' I'm experiencing that. This *is* vital. My son's father and I are separated, he's been missing the baby and wanting to connect about parenting and custody. We never talk. We only send text messages. I don't want to talk, and he doesn't, either . . . but the more we text, the worse it gets. I think we need to meet—face-to-face. Eye contact, like you said. It's vital for our baby. I cried with you in front of everyone because I felt my heart open to love and forgiveness. It's time to grow forward," she shared graciously.

"I feel like there's an even bigger lesson in here about forgiveness, but I can't articulate it," I replied before I thought better and just asked her. "What is it, what's the big lesson?"

"It's about connecting to just being human with each other," she answered. "Forgiveness is simply about aiming in the right direction, you know, and acknowledging we're all equal in our need for love and understanding. It's vital to move forward in life, not backward."

"Is backward really even an option?" I asked in agreement.

"Exactly," she nodded and smiled.

As I walked back to my car, I noticed another friend from the presentation. She was a palliative care practitioner who helps patients prepare for the end of their life.

She walked up to me, "That was amazing."

"I wasn't so sure," I told her, "but for the second part, I had to surrender the notes and just go to the source of information."

"I guess that's how it works best anyway," she added.

"Sometimes, we all need to get out of our own way for healing." I opened my car door.

"That's just so true," she agreed as we turned to hug each other goodbye. Then we both drove away to our next appointments to start our workday.

THE GOOD MEDICINE OF CONNECTION
Medicine Bottle #3

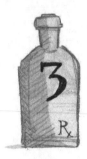

VITAL SIGNS

Energy healing is about connection. We are connecting to parts of our life force that are nonverbal and loving within ultra-consciousness. It's the power of living in the moment that every book on mindfulness and meditation will teach us. But truly, the act of better connection is the path that we are all traveling on. Every path connects us. Connection is considered the most important aspect of being human.

When I connected to the volunteer's energy field, her healing body insisted on making a connection with her adversary. If our bodies are our most resourceful problem solvers, then to bridge from nonconnection to connection is most vital.

Take a moment to connect with yourself through your own consciousness. If you have a mirror available, face yourself not to look *at* yourself but to see *into* your own eyes. Notice what your eyes tell your consciousness. If you do not have access to a mirror, use your clean hands to simply touch your face. Consider your bones, your skin, and your features as parts of you that are *constantly making connections* with the world around you.

By making a connection to listening to your own thoughts, feelings and needs, you are becoming available to connect authentically with others around you. We crave the connections that are good for our health. Getting to know more about yourself and what brings you love, contentment, and peace will allow ease in your connection with every person, idea, and situation you encounter.

Take a moment to list four ways you can connect more earnestly and spend time listening to your own needs, hopes, and desires. See how I started with the first one for you? Now keep going with the rest of the list. Be specific and be true to yourself.

1. I can connect by giving myself *permission* to allow for time and to value the most important connection in this lifetime: My connection to being me.

2. _____

3. _____

4. _____

This is your prescription for the Good Medicine of Connection.

Sudden onset of inspiration is possible. May find an urge to listen more carefully and lovingly when expressing yourself.

chapter 4

HELP

It was a late October afternoon when I closed my eyes and gave up. It was 2001. Personal, political, financial, and professional stressors were at a crescendo. I felt trapped in my own skin. I was suffocated by a collective response to violence with violence in my country, my community, and even turned inward to my heart.

Media messages were packaged in easy logic and justifiable fear, but energetically this surge of fear was even more horrible than grieving the terrorist attacks that surrounded this time in history. I was inundated with anxiety. All escape hatches were blocked by messages of fear on the radio, television, phone calls, and even a peaceful attempt to walk in nature was interrupted with the roaring sound of military planes preparing for war. One particularly anxious afternoon I stayed inside. I watched a fitness tape from the couch. Not having the motivation to even stand up, I watched the workout video, hit the rewind button, and played it over and over again. I felt no relief.

I was newly married with no children. I'd recently lost my job. We'd just moved to a town where I didn't know my neighbors yet. I had nothing to do and no place to go. The fitness tape was clearly not alleviating this sensation of fear and despair. So I turned it off. And there I was. Alone.

How can I escape now? I wondered. I remembered the idea of this thing called meditation. I'd never genuinely tried it. I had no idea where to start, so I closed my eyes and asked: *"Help."*

In about five long seconds I felt a calming presence around me. The sensation was miraculous. I was guided to do something. It felt more like a reminder of something I already knew. That something felt gentle and precise.

"Read this book," was impressed upon my heart. The actual book that I was seeing in my mind's eye belonged to my husband. The book was authored by his friend, Debbie Kane. She was a writer and a painter. She wrote a memoir about how childhood neglect, disability, sexual abuse, and chronic pain informed her wisdom. She transformed her trauma into a richly artistic and love-filled life. But, alas, I had not even read a page yet.

"Read this book," said the voice from my meditation again.

Could I escape my anxiety with the sanctuary of a book? It was absolutely inviting.

We had just moved houses only weeks before, so I had no idea where to find the book. Did it even get packed when we moved?

Still in meditation, I felt a surge of energy that felt like the opposite of the anxiety. I felt lifted up. A bright thought guided me to go to the basement. I stood up from the couch, walked down the stairs, found a stack of boxes, lifted one box, and reached my hand into the next one to grab the exact book, *The Beauty of a Thorn*, almost at the bottom of the box. Suddenly, there it was in my hands.

As if a hardened plaster had begun to crumble from my body cast of fear, Debbie Kane's book was a long chat with a new friend about resilience, suffering, faith, humor, love, and spirit. As soon as I finished reading, I was led to fiction by Steinbeck and nonfiction books by Barbara Ann Brennan, Dolores Krieger, and Alberto Villoldo. I found unread books from college about art history as I dove back into Joseph Campbell's work, and then finally back to *A Separate Peace* by John Knowles about the big tree that still stood right down the street from our new house. The synchronicities were lining up. I read and read and was enriched by all the books waiting for me, aligned in perfect order, for this moment. Before I knew it, December arrived.

I had learned that when all of my attempts to escape, numb, and distract myself from my pain failed, I could surrender.

"Help" was the only word I could utter. It was a whisper and a plea. I read books all day and through the night, and in a mysterious yet efficient and utilitarian way, I found relief in the guidance I was so desperate for.

❧

THE GOOD MEDICINE OF SURRENDER
Medicine Bottle #4

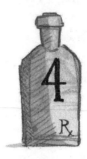

HELP

What are some of your habits that create noise or that block deep listening? Write them down here so they do not operate outside of your awareness:

1. _____

2. _____

3. _____

4. _____

Because one day, these blocks may not be available (like a favorite show, a phone call, or a fitness class) and you will need to ask for help, like I did.

Right now, send the word "help" out as a prayer for yourself.

Now stop. For three full minutes, just listen. What did you hear through your heart and mind? Write it down here:

1. _____

2. _____

3. _____

This is your prescription for the Good Medicine of Surrender.

May experience improved intuition. You may begin to see answers hidden in plain sight. Can be habit-forming.

chapter 5

CAKE ON FIRE

I often work with people seeking the help they have not been able to find in conventional medical or therapeutic approaches. It seems extraordinary that energy healing provides the key to health. But the body's energy field is a common and strong element for everyday health.

"This year I'm practicing receiving for my birthday," my colleague Nora declared in a group email to a few friends, myself included. "I didn't plan a party or a trip. I thought I'd just see what happens when I ask for some help." Her note was festive, brave, and vulnerable. *Good for her*, I thought.

I emailed back, offering Nora a free birthday session of energy work. Two days before her forty-seventh birthday, she sat in my office as we casually caught up about her daughters, her remarkably high-functioning divorce, and her career challenges. She has a gorgeous mane of amber hair and is physically fit because she is a personal trainer. Nora is a cool cat; actually, she is more of a mountain lion. After a few minutes of catching up, we shifted our focus to Nora's health and well-being.

"So what can we work on today?" I asked.

"I don't want this to sound too serious but . . ." Nora began, quieting her voice.

Still smiling, I assured her, "There's no problem with being serious."

"Lately, I keep finding myself thinking that I don't want to go on living," she said.

My mind raced. *This athletic, successful, funny, thoughtful woman . . . what was she saying?* I listened carefully.

"I have this dull despair," Nora said, "and I want to be done with it all. I feel like I want to move on to my spirit and out of this body."

I'm so glad I returned her email, I thought, I had no idea. I took inventory of Nora's every word and intonation. I'm not a doctor, nurse, or therapist, but I work with the health-care community to follow the same rules of safe practice. Nora's safety was my priority now, so I began to ask the questions drafted for me by a psychotherapist:

"Are you feeling hopeless about the future?" I asked.

"Well, no, I have lots to look forward to," Nora exclaimed.

"Have you had thoughts about taking your own life?" I asked.

"Oh God, no, I'd never do that," she said. "It's more of a feeling, despair, or just a desire to move on to something else, more spiritual than just about the physical body." This made sense to me as I took note that she's both a massage therapist and fitness trainer with an expertise in physical anatomy.

"Do you have a plan to end your life?" I continued.

"No, and I wouldn't . . ." Nora said. "I just have to say this because it feels like an imbalance that needs a little tweaking. It's not me, I'm usually upbeat. Well, you know that."

"I do. I know that. But a little tweaking, huh? That's some heavy talk you just landed on for a birthday girl. Perhaps as another birthday gift for yourself, you can book an appointment to talk with a psychotherapist about this, too?"

Nora just nodded and smiled.

"Seriously." I said gently, "I have some great therapists to recommend if you need to find one."

"OK, I promise!" She laughed as she threw her hands over her head.

"OK, let's get you ready for the next forty-seven years," I smiled with her.

Like all my clients, Nora only took off her shoes—in her case, stylish sneakers—and got up on the table. I began my work of scanning her field by moving my hands slowly through the charged air six to twelve inches over her body in the invisible area of her energy field.

While I know through my experience that the energy field exists, even I can be skeptical, because I can't see it. Even though my grandparents were medical doctors who were intimately in contact with the human body's energy, I never heard them talk about this aspect of healing. My working with energy feels totally authentic, while in some ways it feels shockingly out of sync with how I once understood the world to operate. I once thought the world was wholly physical. I thought we could see anything that was real.

When I work with clients, my hands—moving in the space above their body—feel magnetic, gentle currents, and heat shifting. That is life force. My brain is somehow activated to connect meaningfully to images as if my mind is an archive. My clients' energy field communicates to me like we are playing a big game of charades with few rules. Messages and information arise to support the healing process. I believe we are accessing what is known as the "wisdom body." This innate consciousness connects to the physical body, which knows how to heal itself.

Sometimes we actually can see the human energy field. Scientific instruments can measure the bio-magnetic field around the body. This whole planet is pulsing with radio signals emanating from every molecule. Life force is real. In fact, I have found the human body itself is a conscious channeler of life force energy. Our bodies transmit and receive power. And like any other instrument, an occasional tune-up is essential.

At Nora's feet, I sensed a warm tingling sensation signaling to me that her energy was balanced. At her solar plexus, I could feel a restoring force, like a swirl. The strength was unlike the heavy words she expressed when we first began. From her feet to her head, Nora's life force presented as flowing fully and clear.

After several minutes in silence, she was breathing calmly and seemed to be asleep. We had more time in the session, so I wondered what else I could offer her. I remembered her emailed request and meditated on an intention for a spiritual birthday gift. I wanted to connect to her future age of forty-seven—perhaps striking on an insight about the number forty-seven. I kept asking for a birthday message unique to her age. *Forty-seven, forty-seven, forty-sev . . .*

Bam! As if Curly from The Three Stooges with a frying pan interrupted my heartfelt momentary obsession with the number forty-seven, a flash flew across my mind—an image I didn't recognize as a memory.

Startled and a little frightened, I stayed focused on this image. I saw a birthday cake with so many candles that they merged into one flame. It was a cake on fire.

It's impossible to explain how I acquired this understanding, but standing next to Nora, near her right rib cage, I awoke to a revelation about counting time, birthdays, and candles. Along with a frying pan wake-up call and the image of a cake on fire, I had the impression that I was ignorant to want the number forty-seven to reveal itself as a special number. I didn't take it personally, but the impact of being humbled rushed through me. I wanted to bow down. I had asked the wrong question and was getting a clear redirection. I listened intuitively.

The problem is that birthday candles now only represent time gone past. Forty-seven candles do not equal forty-seven years.

I got the impression that this cake-on-fire image also described a new way of counting time. According to Nora's guide, this birthday party cake thing we have been taught all our lives is not actually about marking the years we live. Each candle marks something more bountiful.

In a friendly but unwavering tone, this Frying-Pan-Guide communicated:

You see, life isn't measured by a numbered line. On such an important day as a birthday, why do you humans mark consecutive years? No wonder you find trouble in celebrating.

Pause. And again I saw the cake on fire. I again listened for the message.

Instead, light a candle for each and every blessing you can count. Big blessings, small ones, everlasting, or temporary. Anyone who practices this can set their birthday cake on fire.

Pause.

So go ahead, set your birthday cake on fire.

To complete our session, Nora and I laughed together about the sheer necessity to buy many more birthday candles.

"Who would have thought?" Nora joked. "But of course, don't count the years, count all the blessings of that year."

"I think you may need a bigger cake," I joked back.

As she hugged me, she handed me a hundred-dollar bill. I reminded Nora that this session was my birthday gift to her, but she would not let me hand the money back.

"And aren't *you* supposed to practice receiving gracefully today?" I asked.

With a quick nod, she chuckled. "I said yes to your gift," she said, putting on her jacket, "this is your tip."

One hundred dollars was such a ridiculous tip that I could only shake my head at Nora's explanation. "And maybe you need to get better at receiving, too," she added.

Touché, my friend, I wanted to say. But she was already downstairs.

I never forgot those burning candles covering the top and sides of Nora's large round cake. *Count your blessings and not your years.* She would need many more than forty-seven candles to celebrate her birthday that year.

THE GOOD MEDICINE OF GRATITUDE
Medicine Bottle #5

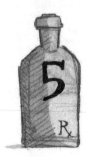

CAKE ON FIRE

I learned from Nora's wisdom that we can enjoy our birthdays more meaningfully by counting our blessings instead of just counting years lived with candles.

As you prepare for your next birthday celebration, start counting your blessings. By years, by days, or by inspiration alone. As much as possible, get into the habit of making your blessings be your measure of life. Right now, take a whole minute and write down as many blessings in your life that flow to your mind.

Ready, set your timer for 1 minute, and go. Start counting your blessings now! Write each one down here:

_____

_____

_____

_____

This is your prescription for the Good Medicine of Blessings.

You will never see your birthday as a mathematical exercise again.
May experience a sudden need to celebrate.

chapter 6

SQUEEZE

Sitting alone in the waiting room, my feet could not quite touch the floor. I was still growing, and my legs were getting longer day by day. I was fourteen years old. Nurses were gathering in the hallway as I swung my legs back and forth and watched the fish tank across from me. My mother's cousin, Virginia, walked in the room and gently said, "She wants to see you," as she took me by the hand.

Grammy Ede was alert and leaning up against a set of pillows. She was pale, her hair not curled, as it usually was, and her hospital gown draped loosely—in sharp contrast to the tailored dresses she wore when she was healthy. She did not have IV tubes coming out of her arms as I expected. This was different. There was nothing on the food tray except a half-filled paper cup of water. Her exquisite posture did not betray her in these last days. She looked like she could just stand up and walk away with me. It brought me little comfort seeing her still so vital knowing why I was there. I held her hand: her right hand in my right hand. I remembered to say, "I love you." She said, "I love you, too," and squeezed a piece of her life back into mine.

I walked back with Virginia, who told me to stay in the waiting area. Alone again, I noticed the fish tank was bubbling with the dull color of murky green. Maybe the fish like it that way, I considered. Perhaps it is the humans who like to see fish in water that's fresh and clear—I'd never seen a fish pond or lake that easy to see through.

I was at the hospital to say goodbye. This was to be the last goodbye ever spoken to Grammy. She was dying, and she knew more about how close she was to death than anyone around her. She was a doctor. She was born in 1899, and eighty-five years later, here she was, losing her life to leukemia. Day after day, the hospital delivered new blood to replace her own, until she told the medical staff to stop. They resisted her request—they didn't want to surrender. She had trained many of those same nurses, and they believed she would get better with fresh blood. We all wanted her to live longer. But my grandmother knew she was not getting better in a fundamental way. She knew how fiercely a failing physical body can hold on at the threshold of life. There was not to be a miraculous turnaround in the coming hours. She planned to say goodbye while she could.

That afternoon, death was still just an abstract idea to me. I watched the fish swim as I remained unbroken by great grief for a few more childhood moments. In the tank, one yellow swimmer played with the bubbling water current pushed from the little pump disguised by plastic seagrass. This swimmer waved its tail fin, furiously resisting the upward surge, and then, as if to surrender, the fish just stopped and ascended among the bubbles. At first, it startled me. *How long had that yellow one been resisting the current's force?* But in the next moment, I saw it swim back to the starting point to begin again—as if playing a game.

In the summertime, only several weeks before, I would race to the steps of the diving board—circling just like this fish. Once there, I'd wait my turn and then take my time as I dug my toes into the porous, sand-glued surface of the well-worn board. I was finally one of the big kids that summer. I knew this because younger kids near the aqua blue slide would turn to look when they heard my heavy spring throwing me upward. Sometimes I'd have a plan for a pike dive or a forward flip. Other times, I would just abandon my form after I sprung into the air to see how my body would tilt and fall back to the water.

Those warm, lazy summer days felt a long distance back in time from this November day.

⁂

At Grammy Ede's memorial service, I sat with my mother, father, sister, and two brothers in the front of the old Congregational church where every wall and pew was painted white, and a balcony wrapped around the sanctuary. Behind me, I sensed the church was full, but I never twisted back to look.

Every other time I came to this church, my grandmother was by my side.

Dressed up with her everyday elegance, she would be greeted with "Good morning, Doc" and "Hello, Doc Hunter." I once asked her if she was bothered by the name "Doc," so casual, like Doc from the Bugs Bunny cartoon. Grammy admitted she didn't particularly like being called Doc, but she told me it helped her patients feel more familiar and comfortable. "That's all that matters," she said. I couldn't possibly imagine that everyone who greeted her by "Doc" was her patient, but perhaps they were.

At Grammy's memorial, the church was full, but all I really remember was that she wasn't there.

⁂

Several years later, when I was home visiting from college, I was massaging my mother's sore shoulder when she mentioned, "You have the same touch as my mother."

"I think I probably have *your* touch, Mom," I argued, "you passed it on to me."

"No, this is different, it's the same touch as my mother. It's unique. You have it."

I didn't quite understand what she was talking about at the time.

THE GOOD MEDICINE OF WISDOM
Medicine Bottle #6

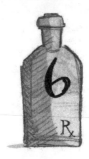

SQUEEZE

If you could imagine holding the hand of someone who loves you fully and sincerely while you are saying goodbye . . . what is your wisdom gift that you want to "squeeze" to this loved one? Maybe it's a different gift for each one. Is this gift for a grandchild or for a friend? Do you believe we can pass our gifts from one person to another?

List three gifts you would share to "squeeze" through your hands to your special person:

1. _____

2. _____

3. _____

This is your prescription for the Good Medicine of Wisdom.

May feel sensations of calm and joy in your heart.
Your sense of deep perspective may grow more quickly than usual.

chapter 7

RAKING

By December 2001, I noticed my body was sore and tense all the time. I needed to move my muscles and get healthier. For stress relief, I started to swim laps but also wondered if massage therapy might be what my body needed. I called a massage school that offered affordable weekly clinics. The year before, I had passed this school twice a day while commuting to the corporate job I had at that time. The school had a big sign posted near the road announcing weekly training clinics and "Massage Clients Wanted" for the students to practice on. On the morning of my appointment, I drove myself to what I remembered to be the location, but found myself at a loading dock behind an abandoned warehouse—precisely the wrong place, even though I thought I knew the location by memory. I was disoriented, and in hindsight, this lack of direction confirmed the effect profound stress had on my brain. I don't remember if I owned a cell phone in 2001. However, I do remember asking a US mail carrier for directions to the massage school and making a call to the receptionist from a pay phone in a booth on the sidewalk.

"You're about fifteen minutes away," said the woman who scheduled the massage clinic.

"Can I still come in?" I knew, more than ever, I needed some stress relief.

"Let me see, if . . . hang on, let me put you on hold."

Waiting on hold, I looked out across the seagrass of the marshes that buffered busy Route One, where parking lots and strip malls seem to float on wetlands. The tall golden grass swayed, offering an elegant backdrop to the undeserving urban sprawl.

"It's too late to fit you in at ten o'clock," the receptionist was back on the line, "but come in for the twelve-thirty clinic after lunch. You'll be seeing Cathy."

It did not matter who I saw. I knew nobody there. I had nothing planned. I booked the new appointment, found myself at the correct location, and just waited in the parking lot for my appointment.

The treatment area was a big room broken into cloth cubicles by white sheets hanging in an elaborate grid to create small private rooms. A soft mumbling emanated from the whole area of student workers and their clients. I felt cautious as I wondered if I had been hooked into a gimmick for a ten-dollar massage. On the other hand, when Cathy approached, her kind blue eyes and confident gait eased my concerns as she introduced herself.

During the first part of the massage, my mind raced as Cathy pushed into a collection of knots in my rhomboid muscles. My shoulders, my neck, and my back were like a plank of oak. Then, the second part of the massage involved an energy healing that I had never experienced before. Cathy was trained in a technique that balances the body's magnetic field. While she was gently touching my shoulder with her right hand and my calf with her left hand, my mind stopped racing.

I felt a quiet that I had not felt before. I was so grateful, I cried. Time shifted as my emotions cleared and my mind remained quiet.

When the session ended, Cathy brought me a glass of water and asked me to sit down. I had already determined that she was some sort of master healer showing up in disguise as a student.

"That was a very powerful session for me," Cathy said, leaning toward me with her hands tucked under her thighs.

I did not know what she meant. Powerful for *her?* I was fundamentally shifted.

"You have a lot of support around you. Do you know that?" she continued.

Through tears and without much thought, I felt another wave of peace when I admitted, "Yes."

Cathy did not hug me goodbye. She explained that she had balanced my energy and she did not want to transfer anything back to me with a hug. I think Cathy could sense I felt disoriented as she cautioned me to drive safely on the way home. She said I might feel a little "out of whack" and I should take it easy, drink only water, and no alcohol or caffeine for the rest of the day. She also invited me to come back to the clinic for the next week.

I did go back. Week after week I was booked with different student therapists because, as part of this school's policy, I could not request Cathy. I got emotionally stronger and more relaxed each time. Then in my fifth week, I was assigned to Cathy again. She brought me back to a state of quiet peace that I had only experienced with her. During our session, I had tears flowing, but I did not feel sadness. I felt the deep relief of knowing there was more to this life and it involved energy healing.

Although I had many friends, a husband, and a large family, I still felt isolated—a feeling I assumed came with being human. I told my husband on our second date that there was only one thing I knew for sure: "You come into this world alone, and you leave this world alone." He never agreed with me on this belief I held so tightly. I did not want him to agree. Nor did I want to be all alone. I just knew I was right. Of course, deep down, I longed to be wrong.

When Cathy told me I had a lot of support around me, I began to feel sensations of comfort colliding with my belief in isolation. Then she said something life-changing.

"I'm not supposed to tell you this; the guides are telling me you're not quite ready to hear this." Cathy talked about "guides" as if she was a news anchor with invisible producers talking into an earpiece. "But I'm going to override them to tell you this . . ."

I may have tilted my head. I may have leaned back. I may have leaned forward.

Cathy told me, ". . . you need to practice raking,"

I thought of the movie *Karate Kid* and the scene with the image of a young student told to practice "wax on—wax off" as part of rigorous martial arts training. The "kid" polishing a car over and over again. In my case I imagined training with dry autumn leaves raking over and over again. I was confused but still curious.

"It's different from what I do here; I practice Polarity. But you'll find a raking class," Cathy said.

"OK," I stumbled to agree, "I have plenty of leaves to rake in my yard." It was late autumn in New England, after all.

She laughed, "Oh no . . . not raking leaves! It's R.E.I.K.I., pronounced ray-kee. It's similar to my work, but not the same principles. It seems to be what you need to do. If you find a Reiki class, you should take it."

Turns out, there was a four-week program a walk from my house for only thirty-five dollars. It was affordable. The class was filled with nurses, police officers, and even a recent military veteran. I guess I only expected massage therapists and some hippie-yuppie types to attend. I think I may have been the hippie-yuppie.

After the first class, I immediately arranged to practice with my friend, Maggie. She had just been diagnosed with cancer at fifty-four years old.

THE GOOD MEDICINE OF GOOD MISTAKES
Medicine Bottle #7

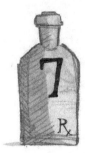

RAKING

Have you ever mistakenly brought yourself to the wrong location? Have you gone to the right place but at the wrong time? If you do not have a time when you made a good mistake, try it. Get yourself lost during your travels to a new destination. Deepen your adventure.

But if you have been in the wrong place before: who or what helped you find your way?

In this chapter titled "Raking," I got a bunch of things wrong, but what appeared wrong added up to remarkable breakthroughs.

List three blessings in your life that at first arrived disguised as mistakes:

1. _____

2. _____

3. _____

List three mistakes that may have yet to blossom into blessings:

1. _____

2. _____

3. _____

Now, write down the lessons that become clear from looking at both of your lists above.

This is your prescription for the Good Medicine of Good Mistakes.

An overall kindness to yourself may settle in after a few days.
Symptoms of inner peace may persist over time.

chapter 8

MAGGIE

Maggie and her daughter Sage were a spirited duet of intensity, honesty, hard work, and humor. I could not imagine them separated. Maggie was going to get better.

Having this powerful energy, I was going to help her beat cancer, even as Sage and Maggie were discussing hospice care. In the hospital, the doctors had just left the room when I arrived. Maggie pressed her head against her pillow and cried. Here we were, all so young, together with the news that there was very little the doctors could do with this diagnosis. As Maggie cried and Sage hugged her, I felt sure she wasn't going to die from this disease.

Maggie was in a bed near the window. In the other bed was her roommate, a woman with yellow eyes.

Liver, I thought.

I'd always known about jaundice because when my brother was a newborn, he needed treatment for jaundice. In contrast, Maggie's eyes were bright; white scleras surrounded her blue irises.

Against the late 2002 backdrop of America's growing war in the Middle East, there was a certain peace in the intimate talk of hospice, medicine, and her hope to overcome cancer. I asked Maggie if I could try some hands-on healing.

"My instructor said I need to practice on someone for five hours before our next class," I said.

"Sure, Hil," she replied as her tears began to settle. I placed my hands on Maggie's head while twisting over the bed's safety bars and the intravenous tubes. I didn't just feel her silky hair but also a warm tingling sensation that dissipated each time I pulled my hands away. Was it magnetic? Was it coming from Maggie?

"Wow, Hil, your hands feel warm like heaters," she said, reaching up to touch my skin. "Why am I feeling all this heat, but your hands *feel* cool?"

"I don't know, but I hope it's helping," I answered. I felt more confident than I sounded.

❧

Three days later, Maggie was still in the hospital getting care for her upset stomach. Sage needed to work all day at her retail job, and asked me to check in on her mom. I arrived and first noticed that Maggie's roommate looked weaker and her eyes were a deeper yellow. I wondered if people died from jaundice. Babies can die from jaundice. So yes, she could be dying I determined as I had the simple thought, *we only have one liver.* The roommate had two visitors sitting next to her in some sort of silent vigil. It was such a somber feeling on that side of the hospital room, I felt protective of Maggie. The grieving and sadness across the room struck me as too sad a mood for her well-being. At this moment, it felt like death was close.

"Hey, Hil, welcome back," Maggie looked up from her crossword puzzles on the tray. The room beeped, buzzed, and smelled of medicines and heavy cleaners. It was a raw hospital environment, but Maggie had made it into her own makeshift office.

Maggie, who was famously organized in matters of materials, swiftly stacked her belongings and pushed the rolling tray to the side. I could have begun care on the area where her cancer originated, but I was first drawn to start at her feet. Cathy, from the student massage clinic, had told me she always begins and ends her energy work at the feet to bring a person's body to a centered and grounded state. A tingling sensation flowed from my hands again. Once again, Maggie commented on the warmth she felt.

More visitors arrived for her roommate. I heard the door gently open and close several times. Greetings were hushed. Someone in the small crowd wept softly. I could not understand their language, but there was an urgency of chatter. The weeping grew. *Maggie's roommate must be dying today,* I thought. Without seeing the group, I could tell there were at least ten visitors. I wondered why Maggie did not even comment on the commotion. She seemed to be profoundly and unusually relaxed. Up to this moment, her hospital stay had not been conducive to resting; yet the action and sounds of chatter on the other side of the room seemed to give Maggie permission to retreat. She was unwinding and I was grateful.

A smiling, middle-aged man stepped halfway around the room's curtain and gestured a hello to me. I was standing with my hands now about a foot above Maggie's torso. I felt embarrassed—as if I was "caught" doing this type of healing. I barely moved except to look up at him. In my new role as an energy worker, I wondered if he would report me back to his group. I felt like an outlier, a rebel, and unsure of how to explain myself. But in that moment of my genuine surprise and his apparent kindness, I felt safe enough to smile back. Our eyes met with some combination of approval and mutual apology. Gesturing, he wordlessly asked if his group was too noisy. I looked at sleeping Maggie and then back at him with a shrug of my shoulders and another smile as I shook my head. *No problem. All is well.*

The man slipped back to his side of the room and immediately the chatter stopped. I feared that I must have miscommunicated some sort of reprimand. *Did he think I wanted everyone else to be quiet for Maggie's sake?* I thought about walking over to explain, but I remained focused on energy healing for another moment. Suddenly, I felt a change. Something in the whole room shifted to a depth of peace I had never felt before. It was such a tangible peace, I decided that it must be the sensation of the group in prayer.

I stayed exactly where I was, careful not to make even the slightest noise of a shuffle. Then the silence broke, but not with talk or even murmur. There was a low harmonious bellow. A chorus of voices igniting into a simple chant— words from another language, and music of a hymn I'd never heard before. The voices sounded like they had sung together many times. The long low notes grew as tenor and soprano voices joined in the song. Even as the hospital room smelled like chemical cleaners and hummed with monitors, it had transformed—as if the air changed color.

This prayer and song was for her roommate, but I hoped Maggie received the overflow of this healing energy, too. My eyes closed as I listened to the voices. This room had become the most sacred hospital room in the world.

Maggie slept soundly, and after another fifteen more minutes of energy healing, I decided it was time to leave, even while the chorus still sang. I was certain the roommate was dying and this must have been a farewell vigil.

Maggie did not wake up as I packed up and put on my jacket. With my back to the cold city window, I felt a sweet comfort among the IVs and emergency buttons and tainted ammonia scents. The room felt blessed. I tiptoed to the door and nodded a thank-you toward the roommate and her visitors.

When I returned to visit Maggie two days later, I found her alone in the hospital room. No roommate was there. That door-side bed was empty.

"Did she die?" I flat out asked Maggie.

"She was discharged yesterday," she said.

"To another hospital?" I concluded.

"No, the nurse said she got better. The other nurses were amazed. Her family came and picked her up."

Maggie was working on another crossword puzzle.

"There were at least five people who came to get her," Maggie continued, "I wish I could get packed up, too. I need to get home. This is no place for me to get better."

That afternoon as Maggie and I visited, we wondered about who the next roommate would be. Maggie reiterated that she didn't want to be around when the next person arrived. I wanted her to say, "go home" rather than "not be around," but I couldn't correct her word choice, and in fact, about twenty-four hours later Maggie was back at her house, too.

THE GOOD MEDICINE OF SONG

Medicine Bottle #8

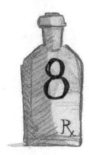

MAGGIE

I heard the song in Maggie's hospital room, but I'll never know the language. Something in this song was healing Maggie's roommate—I wish I knew the words that this small choir was singing.

Imagine what the translation of the lyrics would be? Imagine the quality of the tones and melody. What would you *hope* the lyrics to say?

Write down these possible lyrics in eight lines:

_____

_____

_____

_____

_____

_____

_____

_____

You have created a medicine for poetry and song. This is the song you can sing. The words you can chant to gather yourself. This may even hold someone you love in a healing space.

This is your prescription for the Good Medicine of Song.

May experience impulses to sing out loud and share your songs more often.

chapter 9

"PROUD OF YA"

When Rose started a healing clinic for the oncology unit at the local town hospital, she asked me to join her. Rose was the hospital's official energy healing therapist with a full-time, paid position. Her badge said "Reiki-Oncology." We were students together with shared teachers, and Rose was eager to get me on her team to help cancer patients and their family members.

Twice a month, Rose gathered us, six handpicked practitioners, to hold a healing clinic inside the oncology unit. There were five tables with fresh sheets, and Rose even burned real candles by special permission. The hospital was supportive of this innovative cancer project as Rose created a temporary sanctuary inside the walls of diagnosis, chemotherapy, and radiation. In Rose's enchanted room, five practitioners worked side by side. At the end of each mini session, I thanked the person I worked with and offered my appreciation for our time together.

One afternoon at the clinic, as we ended our session, a patient with a wavy brown wig and soft blue sweatpants asked, "Is it OK if I tell you what I saw while you were working on me?"

I nodded. "Sure."

"I saw white feathers," she whispered.

Suddenly, my heart skipped and my stomach grabbed. Completely disoriented, I felt both a sharp panic in my gut and confusion behind my eyes because this woman was describing what I'd seen. My private, silent, meditative world had been penetrated. I inhaled to gather my nerves. The patient smiled and told me how calm she felt. Behind me, I could hear the routine of sheets being whipped over new beds.

We had almost no time to chat. I wanted to tell her that while I was method-ically bringing my hands to the different energy points over her body and bal-ancing any subtle irregularities in the flow, my mind was daydreaming. I also wanted to tell her that while I was letting my thoughts clear, un-choreographed, I found myself back in time in my grandmother's living room. I recognized the moss-green wool rug and a low-beamed ceiling marking the eighteenth-century reproduction part of her house. It's noteworthy that the ceiling was low because I saw wings. I also saw feathers. Pure white, feathered, muscular wings were so large that they pushed up against the ceiling and surrounded me. The image reminded me of Rembrandt's angels. More than the vision, I felt a visit—I felt my grandmother sending me symbols undeniably hers. The house was hers. This was her living room. Comfort came from her. I recognized my grandmother. The feathered wings were strong, like her personality. It was a gentle impression during the session that had already faded like a dream. If my client had not said the words, "I saw white feathers," I may not have given it a second thought.

With another inhale, and a quick self-negotiation to keep it simple, I burst out in a whisper: "I saw white feathers, too. Wow, they were wings, big wings. I was in my grandmother's house, so I relate these wings to her because, well, she was a doctor, and she would want to help you and me. Something about this all felt familiar, like she was joining me here with you, the way I used to go on house calls with her when I was a kid."

A new oncology patient was approaching my table. Rose quietly handed me a new set of sheets to prep for the next person.

"You seem to have a great deal of support around you. . . ." I told the woman who had seen white feathers, as I unfolded the fresh sheets.

"I know," she said, tying her shoes. "That is amazing. So cool, right?"

"Yes, most definitely, so cool." We said goodbye, and she hurried to the door.

"Thank you," she turned to me one last time.

"No, thank you!" was all I could say.

Cool, I thought, *what an understatement.*

In the days afterward, I became skeptical of this shared and "cool" expe-rience. Factoring in all the clichés that were supposedly "cool," I concluded to myself that this was a coincidence of common thoughts. *White feathers, white wings . . . please!* I was only daydreaming, and so was the woman on the table. Thoughts don't overlap.

꙳

Six weeks later, the random assignments of names and dates for this clinic landed me another chance to work with the same cancer patient. Her familiar smile greeted me with confident eyes that reminded me of our previous moment before I deflated our white feather connection. However, she was the one battling cancer and she had no time for my type of dismissive analysis. With her cancer experience, this oncology patient was more open and flexible in her thinking than I was.

Right before everyone arrived, Rose reminded us of a firm warning from the top administration to not share intuitive insights nor make any elaborate verbal exchanges with the hospital patients. The message was: If we were going to fit this energy healing into the strict culture of health care, we needed to play along—or most specifically, not play—just do the work: focused and silently. Apparently, this order came from the very top administrators who were taking a leap and figuring out if they wanted to keep giving this whole mind/body/spirit thing a try.

This time I got her name. Martha.

During our session, I followed my technique. I scanned Martha's energy field, and then from feet to head, I cleared any energy block that I sensed was obstructing the body's ability to heal.

This time, I intentionally remembered myself back to my grandmother's living room. I invited the white wings to reappear for me. I had forty minutes of silence to explore and directly delve into this ancient practice of hands-on healing that had become second nature to me. All this was wrapped in the sincere intention to help Martha. I tried to concentrate more as I wanted to get back to the wings, but I was being interrupted by something else. Something that created a whole other chasm while I worked. *Why can't I concentrate? Why can't I focus? And what is this odd and unexpected tone I'm taking on around my client? I feel like I'm so proud of her. So very pleased. My heart is puffed with pride, and I just want to give her a big hug and say, "I'm proud of ya, I'm so proud of ya."*

The most confusing part was that although I felt kindness and compassion toward Martha, and indeed I had admiration for her sparkle and strength, I didn't really feel proud of her. It wasn't my place. I couldn't imagine saying, "I'm proud of ya." Moreover, that is not how I talk. I don't tend to have that casual use of "ya," especially while I'm at work. I was so distracted that it no longer seemed to matter what my hands were doing for energy healing. *Great,* I decided to myself sarcastically. I felt very distracted. It had never been so clear to me that I needed help with processing thoughts. It was disorienting to realize I had this distracting thought that didn't even originate with me, and it left me feeling surprised and a little bit scared for my mental health.

Still, at that moment I needed to concentrate; I needed to get back to the wings. But as time ran out, Rose rang a chime to indicate it was time to wrap up our sessions. I was quietly disappointed with myself as Martha opened her eyes and slowly began to sit up. I stepped back to give her space. Sitting on the side of the table, she smiled and thanked me.

"I saw the white feathers again . . ." she beamed.

I hesitated and could only tell the truth, "I didn't quite get there this time, but I'm glad you did. I just need to stick with the energy body and concentrate on that."

"Did any other impressions come through for you? Any other messages?"

Messages? I thought. *Uh, well, hmmm?*

"Not really," I said, noticing my heart started to beat quickly. Fearful I might just blurt out those prevailing words, I recognized that if I told Martha that I was distracted by some circling phrase—"I'm proud of ya"—any of three things could go wrong:

I could sound condescending.

I would be sharing intuition when I've been directed not to share.

It might make no sense to Martha and negate the connection she made with the white feathers from the last time.

All three together were likely to go wrong, but my inner fire and my rapid heartbeat helped me decide to go for it. I decided to take the risk and accept the consequences. I figured that I could handle a reprimand from a hospital administrator, and if necessary, I would try to explain to Martha that I didn't mean to sound condescending.

I began.

"This is going to sound strange because it already sounds strange to me. I mean, I don't want to sound condescending at all, and this isn't really the way I talk . . . but I have a strong impulse to get something out and to say something to you. Is that OK?" I asked.

"Of course," she nodded.

"I feel like I need to say . . ." I hesitated, because it didn't feel like I was using my best judgment here, "Well, I'll just say it. I'm proud of ya. Not proud of you. I'm proud of *ya*."

Martha looked shocked.

"Does that make any sense at all?" I started to dig in or out of this misstep. "I mean, I just felt I should share that, and it's strange because I'd never say 'ya,' I'd always say 'you'—it's just not the way . . ." I stopped talking when Martha put her hands to her face. She was crying. I just waited. Then she lifted her head and smiled with watery eyes.

"I need to tell you something," she said, ignoring the bustle around us. "I got my diagnosis on the day I buried my mother. I found a lump but didn't get it checked out because I was too busy caring for my mom. When she was dying, I told her about the lump because I was starting to get concerned about it. My mom's dying wish was that I'd go directly to a doctor and get it checked out. Before she died, those were some of her last words. 'Get it checked.'"

I listened.

"The day after she died, I had a biopsy, and on the day we buried her, I got the results. I had cancer. She died of cancer."

"Wow, you must miss her so much," I could only imagine.

"You got it, exactly," Martha agreed graciously. "I just wish she was with me during my treatments now. Every morning I take a walk on the beach alone, and I talk to her, sometimes out loud. And this morning, this very morning," she paused, and her chin quivered, "I told her I know that she is watching over me, but it would help so much if I had her approval with everything I'm doing. I told her I needed to know if she was proud of me."

I was speechless.

"And, yes," Martha took a deep inhale and continued, "she would never say 'I'm proud of you.' She'd say it exactly like you said it: 'I'm proud of ya.'"

THE GOOD MEDICINE OF SACRED ANSWERS

Medicine Bottle #9

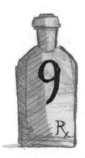

"PROUD OF YA"

Martha told me that she took a walk on the beach every morning. As part of her routine, she would imagine a conversation with her mom . . . a conversation that waited for her deceased mom to answer.

If you took a walk alone every morning, who would you want to be talking to? And what guidance would you ask for?

Would it be someone different every time you walk, or like Martha's walk, would it be one particular person?

Ask yourself, what do I truly need to know? What are the questions deep in my heart that I would ask on my walk?

Ask those questions now. Now listen. Take a full moment. Write down what you may have felt, seen, remembered . . .

_____

_____

_____

_____

_____

_____

This is your prescription for the Good Medicine of Sacred Answers.

May experience miraculous connections. Answers may elate you.

chapter 10

FOXGLOVE

Most people know that foxglove is used in medicine. But here's something less well known: foxglove heals plants as well as people. An old name for digitalis is "Doctor Foxglove," because garden plants near it grow stronger and resist disease.

—Pomona Belvedere, 2009

Once Maggie was home from the hospital, I made a plan to help her. She would have done the same for me. She owned a house one hundred miles away from mine. It was in a forested neighborhood. She was a real estate agent and helped me negotiate the final details before buying our first home. Maggie helped me navigate through zoning laws, survey reports, utility budgets, the rights-of-way, and closing costs. All as a friend sharing her expertise freely with me.

Years earlier, when I moved into my first apartment, my mother asked me to clear out my old bedroom so she could turn it into her office. My small apartment didn't have a place to store all my belongings. Moving out was going to be challenging.

But Maggie met me at my parents' house, and for over twelve hours she went through every piece of clothing, trinket of jewelry, book, and keepsake to teach me how to save what I needed and let go of what I didn't. It was exhausting and emotional. Maggie was gentle yet unrelenting in completing our goal. By the end of the day, I was moved out of my childhood room.

At the apartment, my bedroom was decorated with old wallpaper painted over in deep purple. As bad as that sounds, someone had also made the attempt to paint silver stars to create a "night sky" theme. It didn't work for me.

Renovating this bedroom was crucial to my sense of well-being because I needed, at the very least, a brighter bedroom. I couldn't find respite in that dingy, dark, and barred-window room.

My plan was to remove the wallpaper and paint it a new color. That plan was complicated as I discovered there were nine layers of wallpaper. I peeled and peeled until I was left with a plaster wall of glue and chipped paint covering wood wainscoting.

Maggie had a keen eye for value beneath the surface. She was an antique collector and on the weekends she had her own booth at the flea market. She was innovative and resourceful. When she sensed I was in over my head in the renovation project, she came over with tools and was dressed to work. We began the meticulous job of uncovering the original wood.

Maggie and I worked side by side in that small room. It was a project that tested our patience but deepened our bond. Friends would hear about this endeavor and state the obvious. *"You're renting this place, why waste your time?"* But Maggie never asked that, even as she poured in sweat equity. She saw the value in the care and repair of the room itself, no matter who it belonged to.

When it was done, the wainscoting was smoothly refurbished and the walls were the palest robin's-egg blue. Once complete, the room became a well-earned retreat. Even the bars on the window, solid cast iron, now reflected a sense of protection and ease as I rested or read in this little space.

Without Maggie, it would have been a half-done disaster.

There was no distance that would keep me from Maggie's side as she took on cancer. My experiences with her ability to persevere only added to my resolve that Maggie would get better. Maggie's body just needed a thorough renovation to get past the cancer phase of life. She could outlast and outsmart this disease. She saw potential in lost causes when no one else did. It was my time to help her in any way I could.

But here are some facts that put Maggie at a distinct disadvantage to tackle cancer. When Maggie was diagnosed, she had no health insurance. She was not able to transfer her care to the leading-edge cancer hospitals down the road in Boston. She had remained at the local city hospital. Her doctors would look at her prognosis based on their limited resources. Soon after she was diagnosed, hospice care was referred to assure assistance and comfort in the terminal stage.

To say it happened fast is an understatement. A stomachache turned into a diagnosis, then turned into a prognosis, and she was sent home to manage her quality of life with chemotherapy. That's the hand she was dealt.

Once her treatment started, I drove to visit Maggie twice a week. I was employed at a New Hampshire hospital and my off-hour schedule would easily allow me to take five or six hours for an excursion to help her.

Within a couple weeks, Maggie's soft white hair was gone. Her head was smooth like an eggshell. Her eyes had deepened to a navy blue as she rapidly lost weight.

Her bedroom was a sanctuary with only a large queen bed and a simple dresser. Ever present were three big dogs, Duncan, Lexy, and Otto. They all lived together: A mother, a daughter, and a three-dog pack.

The dogs would greet anyone with a chorus. Her neighborhood was out of the city limits with lots of big trees and boulders. The barking echoed through this suburban forest.

A day after she came home from the hospital, as I drove up her driveway, I heard the dogs barking from inside, but there was no sign of Maggie. I knocked but she didn't answer, so I urgently let myself in. I walked through the unlocked door to investigate. From the kitchen window, to my sincere relief, I could see that she was tending to her late-season garden. I closed my eyes and exhaled. She was meticulous in her methods and I noticed she was digging and planting something. I walked out the back door to greet her.

"Hi Maggie," I said.

"It feels different to work here knowing I won't be doing the gardening in the springtime," she didn't look up.

So defeatist, I thought.

"You're working so hard out here," I said crouching down. She had on her long-sleeve shirt, painting pants, a wide-brimmed garden hat, and heavy work gloves.

"Well, Hil, it's got to get done," Maggie smiled at me. She was planting foxgloves.

I wondered to myself if I had driven down to help her with her garden instead of her cancer. We had set a time but it appeared she had forgotten. Looking back now, that garden had an urgency for her. It was her lifeline.

"I'm tired now anyway," she dusted the dirt from her knees as she stood up. "Where do you want to set up?" she asked.

❧

"I'll put my table in the living room," I said. The room was an uncluttered space with a bay window looking out over more trees in her front yard.

I went inside and set up my table with a fitted sheet and a wool blanket.

When I was ready to begin, I looked for Maggie but she was still in the bathroom.

"I may need a while in here, Hil," she said through the door.

"That's OK," I called back.

"And I'm going to need to get into bed after this," she continued.

"After our session?" I asked.

"No, right after the bathroom," she said.

"OK," I said.

"Yep, OK?" she sounded relieved.

"Of course," and I returned to the living room to put my table, sheets, and blanket back into my car.

When I checked on Maggie about twenty minutes later, she was in her bed looking so much smaller without her hat and garden gear.

"It's nice to visit you at home instead of in the hospital."

"You said it," she agreed.

"Is it OK if I try some hands-on healing on you while you rest?"

"That's what I was hoping for," she said.

"Good." I started by scanning her abdominal area with both hands. The air above her pelvis felt cold and heavy. I imagined breathing in sunshine and being an antenna to get that sunshine energy to her cancer.

The session truly began when I felt my hands tingle with warmth. With my only intention to increase her connection to life force, I focused on her solar plexus, heart, head, and feet. Over and over, I studied the flow of energy that day. The cold air became warm and the heaviness dissolved. She was asleep when I left her house.

This would become our new visiting routine. Sometimes Maggie was already resting in bed, sometimes she was in the kitchen, and most often, she was tending to the dogs. The garden was set for the season. Snow was coming soon, but I was certain Maggie would see the springtime.

THE GOOD MEDICINE OF PLANTING

Medicine Bottle #10

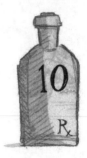

FOXGLOVE

If you were to have an insight into your seasons ahead and thought you may not be "here" a year from today, what would you plant to bloom without you? Would it be an idea, a gift, a letter, a flower, a tree, or something else?

Imagine this world without you in it, and plant something beautiful today.

Write down three seeds planted that can grow onward. Was it the seed of an idea, a dream, a hope, or a vision?

1. _____

2. _____

3. _____

This is your prescription for the Good Medicine of Planting.

You may discover a resilience that is both perennial and joyful.

chapter 11

APOPTOSIS

Apoptosis, or programmed cell death, evolved as a rapid and irreversible process to efficiently eliminate dysfunctional cells. A hallmark of cancer is the ability of malignant cells to evade apoptosis.

—Hanahan D, Weinberg RA[1]

Once in a while I find myself understanding a beautiful order connecting nature to healing the body. The elusively profound message of "letting go" flows though themes of addiction, trauma, mental illness, and disease. My very best lesson about letting go was taught to me by a fallen maple tree.

When I was a child growing up in New England, I thought all trees that weren't evergreens died in September and October and came back to life in April and May. Later in life, I associated the four distinct seasons with the seasons of a long life.

Birth connects with spring.

Summer connects childhood into adulthood.

Autumn is the aging process.

Winter is the end of life.

One day in October, I stopped on a bridge to admire the crimson glow of red leaves from a tree collapsed in the river. A windstorm had struck the night before, and a large maple tree in full brilliance dropped directly into the water.

---

1 Hanahan, D., and R. A. Weinberg. 2011. "Hallmarks of Cancer: The Next Generation." *Cell 144:646–674. PMID: 21376230*

Above, the sky was clear, and the reflection doubled the magnificence of this tree. It had fallen and was dying, but just like the other trees expressing the cycle of life, I thought, its beauty was majestic.

Every day that week I walked to that dying tree. My route included the campus of Phillips Exeter Academy beyond writer John Knowles's *Separate Peace* tree and into the woods beyond the football fields. My walk to the river begins with brick paths and storied architecture, then flares open to the library designed by architect Louis Kahn. I passed a massive concrete building actually named Love Gymnasium, then into the manicured fields, along the winding river and into the acres of forest trails. The *Separate Peace* tree was far behind me now, but these walking trails held the spirit of Knowles's title.

Each day, I returned to the river while the stellar beauty of red leaves became more and more submerged. The yellow and orange foliage from the standing trees framed the whole colorful vista.

My childhood understanding of the cycle of life and the cycle of the seasons was now being affirmed in front of my eyes.

And as autumn often pulls us back to work indoors as the summer light exits, I took too long to return to the river the next week. All around New England the leaves were down. Snow had nature's permission to descend now. When I returned to the fallen maple tree, the air was cold, but the river still flowed without a wisp of ice. Below the bridge, yellow leaves had pooled into a boat-shaped inlet: stopping, swirling, and sometimes escaping. Standing above the banks were clean, gray branches achingly gorgeous in their complex geometry. Every tree is a great balancing act against weight and wind and height.

And yet, I noticed this fallen maple tree in the water did not drop its leaves. The branches clung to brown and dry chattering leaves. This tree was dead. Above me, the bare trees were alive.

The silhouette of bold trunks and bare branches seemed, all at once, vital and confident for the next season of snow. And, all at once, I understood that dropping leaves is an act of living, not dying.

I stood on the bridge over the water and studied this fallen tree. This collapsed tree represented a more accurate death image. The dry brown leaves stayed attached because a leaf cannot drop without an active life force. The dropping away of foliage is called apoptosis—the same name as the medical term for actions of living cells opening up and letting old matter fall away.

That autumn, the dying tree in the river taught me about the practical wisdom of letting go. Apoptosis is the healthy nature of programmed death. I learned that what we do not release can become cancerous and burdensome. I would bring this lesson to my healing practice.

THE GOOD MEDICINE OF LETTING GO
Medicine Bottle #11

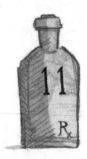

APOPTOSIS

Become aware of your hand and clench your fist while asking yourself, "What do I grip too tightly in my life?" Now write your answer here:

_____

_____

_____

_____

_____

Now open your hands and stretch while looking at your answer above.

I walked over a bridge and discovered the symbol of letting go. Imagine yourself on your own special bridge that is leading you to a new place. What is your symbol for letting go?

Let your mind write freely as you release the grip of whatever you are holding on to. It is the definition of health to be able to let go *over and over* again.

Write it all down here:

_____

_____

_____

_____

_____

_____

_____

_____

_____

_____

_____

_____

This is your prescription for the Good Medicine of Letting Go.

May be surprised to feel more clarity and more energy. Problems may drop away.

chapter 12

MURPHY

I had only known Murphy for about three minutes when he told me he doesn't believe in God. In the fourth minute, he described his unwavering belief in an infinite connection to the cosmos back to the very beginning of everything.

Then Murphy told me with his square shoulders and a glimmer of pride, that he has no fear of dying. He understands death as the body just dissolving back into the same vibration of energy born from the big bang itself.

Murphy said, "I'm not afraid to die, but it's not my time."

I began at his feet and shins to tune into a warm, vibrant buzz. It was not the depleted or tired life force that I sometimes associated with cancer. A magnetic pull across his upper body eventually had me hovering at his right shoulder.

In the metaphysical body map, the right shoulder locates the Akashic records. In charting a body's energy system, these records are the accounting of the history of both our past lives and our soul's journey. It is like a library for every molecular memory, or like a gathering place for all our ancestral knowledge. It is also the location of his arm and his shoulder; simply where muscles and joints come together. I considered all this as I focused on healing his body.

As I concentrated, an annoying distraction fell into my head like an unwanted daydream. At first, I did not recognize it as anything more than an odd but passing thought. But the distraction remained. Over and over. Not just a thought, but a memory laced with heavy emotions.

I want to kill myself. I remembered the words so clearly. He was twenty-one years old crying on the phone, and I was eighteen. My boyfriend of four long-distant years had just been driven to the bus stop by my parents after they walked in on us half-naked in my bedroom. We were in love and stealing away for a moment. But we lost track of our time and our setting. He was immediately kicked out of my house and sent back to his home five hours away on a bus.

The memory was sudden and tangibly uncomfortable. A personal low point in my life and one that I did not want to recall. It was tapping into an emotional element that was even heavier than my previous recollections of that event. I felt the most profound despair. The emotions were overwhelming. Like a punch in the stomach, the despair was fraught with humiliation and abandonment. Those were the only words I could find. *Humiliation. Abandonment.*

"I'm trying to get clear about this area," I said. I was still standing near Murphy's shoulder.

"I don't have any trouble with my arm," he relayed.

"It's more of an emotion, a weight that feels like an incredible burden. I almost want to walk out of the room and splash water on my face to wake up from it."

Murphy, of course, hadn't a clue how this was part of a healing session. But I sensed he trusted my earnestness and he remained curiously involved.

"How so?" he said efficiently with a slight Maine accent.

"A humiliation and a sense of abandonment . . . a deep sense," I told him.

It seemed big enough to be related to his cancer, but I was not sure at all.

"That's not really part of me. I have a beautiful family," he said, "and I don't feel humiliated ever, not overly proud, but not humiliated, either."

I let it go and my hands moved away from his shoulder area.

Once I spoke it out loud, the ghost of this memory let me go, too. There must have been trapped energy now released.

I finished up our hour with notes to include the emotional impressions, and I got permission to share my notes with his referring doctor.

As a single session, I hoped I had done enough energy work to support his cancer battle.

The next week, Murphy was back. Apparently, I was to learn, Murphy does his homework.

"I remember," he said.

"What's that?" I asked. It had been a long full week for me since we worked together.

"The humiliation. *And* the abandonment."

"Oh?"

"I was never a good reader or writer," Murphy began. "Only did school until I was in eighth grade. But I liked this girl. And that was a big deal at that age. We were at a party, and I never kept my wallet in my pocket, because I didn't have enough padding back there. Too bony, if you know what I mean. So I guess my wallet was in my jacket hanging by the door and I had a note written for the girl in it. One of my friends' little brothers grabbed the note out of my wallet and said, 'Want me to read it? Want me to?' He was talking to me, but I wasn't really paying attention to what he had in his hand, so I shrugged and said, 'it doesn't matter to me.'"

Murphy leaned toward me and then looked away toward the only window in the room.

"Yeah, humiliating and isolating," his eyes watered as he was visibly upset.

"How so?"

"I left the party," he said.

"Kicked out?" This was starting to make sense.

"No, I left, and I didn't grab my coat or wallet. I just left. See, that boy read the note about how much I liked this girl, and it made no sense because I couldn't really write well. I had no real education. And the girl was there with her friends. I really liked her. They all laughed. I just couldn't stay."

"So you left."

"I left." Murphy said.

I understood the humiliation, but I asked, "What about the abandonment?"

"Those were all my friends there. That was all I had. You know that age. I was alone for quite a while after that. Took a long time to recover. Parties like that were everything in those days," Murphy exhaled a sigh for his childhood.

"So you found it," I said.

"I found it, and you were correct—a heavy memory I'd just as soon forget."

"But your body remembered."

"Indeed it did."

The next week, at the same time, Murphy had more to report on humiliation and abandonment.

"My mom was divorced. My dad was gone, never knew him, but my mom was great on her own. Truly. And I had a best friend up until I was nine years old."

I let him continue.

"His name was Garrett, and we played all the time in the neighborhood, my house, his house. Terrific friends," he began.

I listened as I put new sheets on the table.

"Then one perfectly normal afternoon his mom opened the door and said, 'You're not allowed in, your mom is a tramp, and you just can't play over here anymore.'"

I thought Murphy was joking by the lilt in his voice. But he wasn't. He was tearing up. I stopped and sat down with him.

"After almost ten years my mom wanted to marry again and she started dating this man . . . and it's a small town. Very strict Catholic town back then, and she was shunned. And so was I."

"Humiliation and abandonment. For sure," I agreed.

"Yep," he said.

"What a loss for you as a kid."

"Yeah, that's how I remember it. I was lost."

The next week Murphy arrived prepared again. Before he sat down, he looked at me and said, "I guess I should tell you how I was beaten up by my stepfather. Not a good man. I wasn't perfect, either. But I was just a kid, and he wasn't good to any of us."

I felt heartbroken.

"I tried to protect my sister and brothers, but I had to go," he said.

"You ran away?"

"To the war," he laughed without humor. "I was only seventeen years old and I was small for my age, but I needed to go far away because I needed to belong somewhere. I wanted to be a soldier with other soldiers. It made sense. It really did."

"How'd you enlist at seventeen?" I asked.

"I lied, I just said I was eighteen. They never told me my documents were wrong. They took me, and I went."

"Where'd you go?"

"That's the funny part—it was kind of an abandoned post. I joined for camaraderie, but I was posted in the most remote, isolated place with only one other soldier who slept the opposite shift. We manned a nuclear warhead on a Korean mountain."

The next week, Murphy said his father left him as a three-month-old baby.

"That must definitely count as some kind of abandonment," he reflected, "even though I was too young to notice."

"I think so," I agreed.

At the following session, Murphy told me how he was never furious at his father.

" I understand my father left me because he was heartbroken."

I felt myself frown and tilt my head, suddenly protective of Murphy.

"I had a three-year-old baby sister—well, actually she was older than me—but she died when my mom was pregnant with me. I think my dad was afraid to love another baby again. So he left all of us."

The next week Murphy mentioned that throughout his whole childhood his mom told him that his father was dead. But one day when Murphy was packing for deployment to Korea, his mom walked into his bedroom and told him his dad was alive and lived in Hawaii. She thought it was serendipitous that his military flight stopped in Hawaii, so she told him the truth. She suggested that Murphy should look him up.

"Holy what? How on earth did that go?" I was shocked for him.

"Oh, as expected . . ." he crossed his arms and looked out the window.

"Which was . . .?"

"I met him, and my dad and I drove around the island like a couple of tourists. Didn't have much in common. I only had six hours on the island."

"That must have been incredible. You thought your father was dead and then you got to see him on your way to war?"

"Yeah, it was interesting but not incredible. The visit was long enough," he said.

"Did you keep in touch?"

"He sent a couple of letters and then that was it. Wasn't much."

"Can you imagine?"

"Imagine what?" he uncharacteristically snapped back.

"Leaving your kids like that."

"Oh God no, I just don't relate to him or anyone who'd just leave a child like that," his anger was palpable and, I considered, well justified.

"So that's it," I acknowledged the weight of all the memories he had excavated.

"Yeah, I think that's everything," Murphy said softly.

"You found humiliation and abandonment in your history," I reiterated.

"Took me long enough."

"But we got there, and now how do you feel?" I asked.

"I feel better," he noticed, "and we did get there."

"Good. Let's see, what else comes up today?" And we began the energy work again.

THE GOOD MEDICINE OF BRAVERY
Medicine Bottle #12

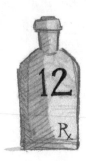

MURPHY

As a courageous young soldier, Murphy was packing his bag to head to war. But in his battle with cancer, he needed to unpack the burden of humiliation and abandonment that was hiding in his body.

Another person may not have looked any deeper beyond the first reaction of denial. Murphy had extraordinary bravery. Week by week, he slowly and methodically unpacked any memories of humiliation or sensations of abandonment.

For Murphy it was "humiliation and abandonment" and I, as his practitioner, was brave enough to speak up and share all the unpleasantness packed away.

Murphy was brave to believe we could unpack humiliation and abandonment together. He trusted the message and stayed curious as he unpacked any obstacles to his health.

What are some blocks that are keeping your wounds from healing? How deeply are they packed away? Murphy was gentle and protective of himself as he unpacked his issues week by week. Be gentle, too, as you quietly and honestly ask yourself: What do I need to unpack? List two possibilities here:

1. _____

2. _____

Murphy also didn't do this alone. List who you would want by your side to help you calmly unpack your bags and burdens.

_____

_____

_____

_____

_____

_____

This is your prescription for the Good Medicine of Bravery.

Expect sudden and impactful self-awareness.
May experience bursts of courage and accelerated healing.

chapter 13

OWL

It would be easy to never notice Marc's sage-colored house. Across the street is a big wooden statue of a bear advertising a campground. That's my landmark for his driveway. That bear also is a landmark for a magical, healing place. It stands as a testament to the dirt roads and their well-built homes that once connected these northern seaside towns from Boston to Maine.

Marc welcomes me through the side entrance into the warm kitchen anchored by a farmer's table. This antique Cape Cod style house holds a sense of authentic history inherent to the work Marc does here.

In this kitchen I have sat with Marc for some of the most critical head-cracking moments of my growth. These are the times when I willingly invited a healer to shake my soul and clear my karmic canvas.

Beyond the kitchen, there is an entryway to his healing room. The wide pine wood floor, covered with scattered handwoven rugs, creaks as I step toward a big couch that holds me like Alice in her teacup. On the walls are images of wolves and feathers and bones and drums and colorful paintings that all seem to huddle around Marc.

This is the room where I took my first shamanic journey from a futon mat in the center of the room. As I began, I could hear through the windows the sound of cars blindly passing this magical place at fifty miles per hour.

Inside, Marc and I were stationary but traveling. We were moving at the speed of time, memory, and collective consciousness together in this session. He described a place called the Lower Earth, an idyllic place where humans can only briefly visit. From how I understand it, this is where nature's intelligence dominates without the overlay of the human ego filter. It's only "lower" the way the heart is lower than the brain. It's rich and subtle. It's the fairytale dreamed over and over by children of every culture. It's the place where water-falls talk to squirrels.

The old word for journeying to Lower Earth is "imagination." The new word hasn't arrived for me yet. Perhaps it never wants to have a word—but to journey to this world requires an unquestioning commitment to slithering out of the limits of the daily mental structures that usually constrain adults.

On this particular day, I didn't need to fully understand the Lower Earth because Marc, as a shaman, journeyed *for* me. In this other world, through guided meditation, he brought me to a mystical location to find answers to the questions I could barely articulate. Like a dream, I was suddenly there, stand-ing in a grassy field. There were no horizons and no maps. In my half-awake state, I was free and vacant all at once. I could still feel the mat beneath my resting body but almost nothing else.

Forgetting I wasn't alone, Marc's voice startled me. "Grandfather asks me to find out why you're not having children."

"Who is Grandfather?" I found my voice back from my dream to ask. I wondered how he could possibly know what I was grappling with? *Why would he ask this?*

"Who is asking this?" I spoke.

"A spirit guide, my dear, who is wondering about your choices."

Now here's the thing about this dreamlike state of trance that Marc had taken me on: my answer surprised *me*. If I wasn't standing in an imaginary green field, in a meditative-trance-like state, I could have crafted a rationalized response. Perhaps more clever and probably less honest, I'd have a grand expla-nation for the childless adult life I was planning. Instead, I heard myself say:

"I have my children."

"Oh really," the playful part of Marc engaged with me. "Where are they?"

"Not born, but safe and loved." I spoke calmly.

"So you just imagine them to exist, but not here?" he said.

"They are safe," I whispered confidently.

"So you don't have any children because the children you have are safe?"

"Yes." I felt calm and delighted by myself. I hadn't ever spoken this out-loud. In a flash, I could see how this shamanic journey was helping me create a comfortable framework to heal my life. I had not given much thought to why I had not craved children like some of my friends. I was married, settled, and the timing *could* be good for childrearing. But it was not good timing, and it would never be. Now I knew why.

"Yes, that's it," I repeated as my body rested into a deep relief.

"Grandfather tells me to say you are arrogant," he said in the gentlest fashion. "This is arrogant to think your fear is keeping your children safe."

It was arresting to be called arrogant, but I was too relaxed to fight. Marc was correct. It *was* fear.

"I have a right to not have children," I argued to this Grandfather Spirit with my eyes still closed.

"Yes you do, but this reasoning originated from your fears. You are not protecting anyone; you are just choosing to not live your life. What is this fear?"

"I was scared all the time as a child," I admitted. "I can't defend this world as a safe place."

The shaman surprised me with a little laughter. "Ha!"

What's so funny? I wondered on the verge of tears, arguing from a lifelong belief born from a promise I made to myself. I promised I would not subject my children to the horror of wars, broken bones, and absolutely everything in between. *This is my journey and I'm playing it this way.* I dug stubbornly into my thoughts.

And then Marc asked me to breathe. As he pushed the heel of his hand to my solar plexus, I had no choice but to exhale. Then I took a deep inhale. I felt exhausted by this brief argument about fear and children and childhood. I just wanted to fall asleep. Marc instructed my breathing. The journey had barely begun.

"Where are you?" Marc woke me.

My eyes jumped open, "I was flying with an owl."

"Yes, I know—you are with Owl now. See the world through Owl's eyes."

I closed my eyes again.

"How do I do that?" I asked.

"Where are you now?" he asked back.

"It seems that I'm in my yard, but I'm looking down at the snow—it's crunchy snow. Not good for snowmen." I felt far away from the wooden floor that was right beneath me.

"How old were you when you lived here in this yard? Where is this yard you're in?" he guided.

"It's my yard now, where we live now. I'm in the backyard of my house," I answered.

"Good, good, good," I heard Marc say. "What do you see?"

"It's night, and the windows glow warm with light—it feels welcoming, like I want to come in from the cold."

"What are Owl's eyes showing you?"

"That this is my house, this is my home, and it's warm and safe here."

🦉

Two months later, on a January day when the icy snow was crunchy to step on, I saw an owl perched in the same tree as I saw in the journey with Marc. Exactly as I had seen it, this big owl was facing our house. I had never seen an owl in our yard before or since then. It stayed for almost an hour. I watched to see the moment when the owl would fly away. I wanted to witness the wings spanning. But this owl stayed on the branch looking toward my house. It was only when I looked away to pour a glass of water that the owl disappeared from view. It was gone, but I never did see it fly away.

🦉

By April, I was pregnant with my first child.

THE GOOD MEDICINE OF AWE

Medicine Bottle #13

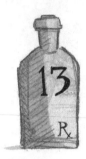

OWL

My experience with Marc and the owl in my yard was awesome.

With help and what seemed to be mystical intervention, I was brought past obstacles of fear back to my heart's wisdom.

Allow yourself to live in awe for a moment. It's deceptively simple. Observe this moment and feel equality with everything in your world. Feel with your senses, feel with your emotions, and even feel your thoughts. Follow all this until you feel awe. Be honored. Honor everything. Now take notes.

List three elements in this moment that inspired you.

1. _____

2. _____

3. _____

And to become even stronger, list three more:

1. _____

2. _____

3. _____

This is your prescription for the Good Medicine of Awe.

Life will become a journey. May notice more wild birds around you.

chapter 14

PEARL

It was the type of party where I could wear fancy heels at noon in December. A ladies' luncheon was hosted for my friend turning forty years old. Bonnie Jean is a most-cherished gem of a person. She is a tapestry of kindness, wit, insight, patience, humor, and phenomenal artistic talent. She's the type of person I could smother with friendship. She's easy to love. That day at her party, the room pulsed with pure celebration.

Everyone else had already turned forty except me. I was feeling a little left out. The rest of the women all seemed to know each other better and doted on the birthday girl. Residing confidently to the side of the crowd and joyfully observing the action was Pearl, the birthday girl's mother.

Pearl is a superstar of energy. I usually could not catch up with her. She dances, plays piano, and has quick humor . . . even when she's not onstage. Her petite dancer's body could wear anything including the 1960s-era classic A-line dress she wore in honor of her daughter's birth. She is often the life and zest of any gathering, but today, her quieter, observant mood allowed me to float over and strike up a conversation.

"Hello, Pearl, happy birthday to you, too. I think mothers need more credit on this anniversary of birth, don't you agree?" I leaned against the wall, so our heights matched eye to eye. I was eight months pregnant.

"Oh, I remember it like yesterday," she swept her hand across the space between us to indicate the ease in which life flows. With breezy comfort, Pearl was a model for active longevity. I wanted to believe that life can be as smooth as her hand motion described.

"Have you been dancing lately?" I ask rhetorically.

"Like this?" Pearl shimmied her feet, did a little hip twist, then winked.

I laughed and lost my words—I was out of my league as usual around Pearl. I was striking up a conversation with a rock star at intermission.

Then graciously, Pearl asked if I'd been dancing lately. I felt my face flush. *How did she know that I was once a dancer?*

"Uh, not lately" I admitted. "But I miss it."

"Well you must be doing something you love . . . you know you must," she sipped from her punch glass but kept her eye contact on the question. Pearl lived vigorously, and advocated for it, too.

OK, I'll tell her what I've been up to.

"Actually, I've found something I love to do recently. It's a little out there, I know," I hinted.

"Well that's not a bad thing," she nodded, and with the slightest hand signal encouraged me to go on.

"I've been studying healing since I was a kid, but I'm excited that I learned a new technique—it's considered by some to be a new modality but also, by others, an ancient practice —a type of healing with hands."

Pearl looked unfazed—I thought she was hunkering down for a boring explanation that had nothing to do with stages, sparks, or waltzes. So I decided to dazzle her with a story.

"I've been working with the oncology department at the hospital . . . we work with several patients over the course of an hour. One woman said she felt tingling all across her abdomen during her session—even when my hands were on her feet! Turns out, her abdomen was the location of her tumor. I had no other way of knowing that. It was fascinating."

Pearl took another sip.

"And I also tried it on my friend's cat, Misty, who was sick in her bed and not moving for days. After five minutes of connecting with this energy buzzing in my hands, she jumped off my lap and pranced away—her people were amazed and I was, too. The cat pranced away when we thought she couldn't walk." I was animated. I wanted Pearl to know I was doing exciting things.

"Oh I know, I've heard of it," she said quietly with a calm nod.

"Yes? Oh good, because not many of my friends have. It may seem like I'm crazy."

"Never ever worry about anyone thinking you're crazy. Life's too short."

I considered how elegantly Pearl tried to change the subject while imbuing more wisdom.

"Energy as a healing medicine is starting to get better known though. They're allowing it at some hospitals now. Right up in Portsmouth was the very first hospital to offer it officially. And I've heard Columbia University is pioneering a new program for inpatients," I jabbered—possibly being a little too enthusiastic. Then I decided to slow down.

"Wait, so, how did you know about energy healing? Did you have a session at a hospital or something?"

"Oh, no dear, I practiced this all myself a long time ago," she suddenly seemed uncharacteristically sad.

Honestly, I thought she was confused.

"You did hands-on healing?" I floated my hand back and forth like I was practicing right there.

"Yes," she understated.

"Around here?"

"No, as a nurse's assistant in the military."

Now I was really impressed. I think I could only tilt my head in curiosity.

The other guests circled the luncheon table as fresh warm soup in hand-crafted bowls waited at each seat.

"When were you in the military?" I asked urgently, but attempted to be calm.

"The war, my dear, in the war," she said. That's really the way Pearl spoke.

"You mean *the* war?" I calculated, "World War II?"

"Oh yes, all the nurses did this energy type of healing for the soldiers. We helped the enemy as well as our boys, of course. We all did it back then—it was just what we did."

What? Huh? United States Military and hands-on healing? My questions were mounting but my time was up. Pearl was swept off to her seat at the head of the table. I was sure I would learn the history of military, nursing, and energy healing another time. I had so many more questions for Pearl.

The luncheon was homemade deliciousness with an utterly delightful spirit of celebration. Chatter and laughter rose between delicacies. When it was time to say goodbye, Cate, one of Bonnie Jean's friends, commented on my visible pregnancy. I was due in a month. Cate pulled me aside and mentioned that she has birthed eight children.

"Can I give you some advice about labor?" she asked.

"Sure!" I agreed. *God, please, No!* I silently pleaded. I'd heard more labor horror stories in the past month . . I hoped to forget them all before my water broke.

"Everybody says it's tough," she read my mind, "but I say, 'Have fun, Enjoy it!'"

"Enjoy . . . you mean . . . labor?"

"Yes!" she curled her arm flexing her bicep like the blue scarfed woman in the World War II posters, "It's an athletic event, it's *the* athletic event. You're ready for it. Have fun!"

"OK," I strained a smile, looking at the other luncheon women for confirmation but getting none. "I'll try to remember that."

"Own it," she insisted. "It's truly a sport. Enjoy your labor! I'm telling you, it's not easy, but it's a lot of fun. I know. I had eight!" Cate had burst into full coaching mode.

"Can I take you with me to the hospital?" I was starting to be convinced I needed more of this woman in my life.

"You won't need me," she assured me as I walked out the door.

I turned to Bonnie Jean and gave her a parting hug.

"Goodbye and thank you," I waved to the remaining guests. Pearl stood back and offered me a knowing wink.

THE GOOD MEDICINE OF COMPASSION
Medicine Bottle #14

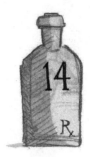

PEARL

Have you been assigned an enemy? In your culture, in your village, at work, or even in your family?

Can you describe your enemy?

Now ask yourself, if your enemy was wounded, would you care for them?

Pearl stopped short of sharing her full story with me. What is the story that you would like to imagine Pearl told me as an assistant military nurse in wartime, caring for our enemies? Who was the enemy? What care did the enemy need?

Write it down here.

_____

_____

_____

_____

_____

_____

Sometimes very good people care for their enemies. And that is very good energy.

This is your prescription for the Good Medicine of Compassion.

Authentic connections may form spontaneously. May smile, laugh, and dance more frequently.

chapter 15

VASILOPITA

In the same way Murphy's very first words to me were about God and the cosmos, I have many clients express their religious beliefs concerning their own healing. Part of the work I do could be described as hands-on healing—and spiritual health is a crucial part of ancient traditions from all around the world.

I have clients who assert their strong *opposition* to any formal religious references to healing for a range of reasons. I also have clients *request* prayers for healing in the name of their religion and their understanding of God.

I would never deny following any such request or oppositions in the name of healing. I understand that it is my job to facilitate the body's innate ability to heal, including the spiritual resources that are grown from everybody's own beliefs and needs for spiritual boundaries.

Adela has a sweet, float-through-the-room type of personality. She is actively spiritual, and smart about other people, their stories and their struggles. As my client, I would assess that Adela sees her world as sacred in its daily happenings. She booked a session with me right after the new year.

"In the Greek church," she explained, "we bake a loaf of bread at the beginning of each year. We put a coin in it and, for my family, our tradition is to cut a slice for every member of the family."

"What kind of bread?" I asked.

"It's called vasilopita, I think because of the basil. It doesn't matter," she said, shaking her head playfully at me.

But I was already considering how basil bread would taste dipped in olive oil.

"What matters," she continued, "is that we always cut the first piece for baby Jesus—it's part of the tradition."

"OK, got it," I stopped thinking about olive oil.

"This year, on the first slice, we hit the coin. That means this is the year devoted to Jesus."

"Huh, very interesting. That's a tradition I've never heard of." I was intrigued.

"It's just something we do," again she waved her hand playfully toward me while adding, "but I tell you all this because I want this session with you to be dedicated to this year of Jesus."

I told her that I could try that. I'm familiar with the healing tradition of Jesus. I was, after all, brought up as a Protestant (mother's family) along with a devoted family of Catholics (father's family.) I have a deep respect and reverence for the Jewish culture, too. I'm not well versed in Buddhism, Hinduism, or Islam but I'm inspired by the idea that in world religions there are healing arts rooted with love and faith in each tradition.

"I've been asked to do this before, " I told her.

I told Adela about the time a colleague, an acupuncturist, booked a session with me. I thought this client would be very comfortable with hands-on healing as a fellow practitioner. However, she didn't want me to do any energy healing with her unless I did so in the name of "Jesus Christ Lord Our Savior." If she hadn't been my colleague, I may have asked more questions or even attempted to draw clear boundaries between the nature of my work and her beliefs. But it turned out, saying the prayer she requested brought ease to our process and her body was clearly receptive for healing. In fact, her health issue had been a problem for over twenty years but while following the "homework" I gave her after her only session, she had a big healing event, and her entire issue was resolved within two weeks.

I respect and honor the religious and spiritual needs of my clients. Having a connection with a spiritual source is one of the cornerstones of health.

Per Adela's request, I started by asking out loud for this session to be guided and blessed in the spirit of Jesus. Adela whispered thank you.

I had barely started to work at her feet when a wave of pink light flooded the session. It's not that the room looked pink. Not that at all. There was just a presence that felt, well, pale pink. It's odd to describe a feeling as a color, but that's what it was.

I let the energy of the room flow to me and through me. Adela was deeply relaxed, and her breath was steady. I repeated the prayer as I dedicated my work to trust her spiritual body.

Suddenly the pink light carried more than just color, it brought a message: *First, let forgiveness in, then let gratitude in, then begin your prayer.*

I felt a very literal sense of a plan forming. This was the beginning of a list of some sort. So concise, not at all like I usually intuit, but clearly arranged for Adela. I did not speak it; I took a pencil and wrote down those exact notes.

I brought my hands back to her body, this time near her shoulders, and another equally calm message flowed in.

With all prayer, hold the intention for miracles. Let miracles in.

I stayed quietly with the message and then turned to write again. Then, back to the hands-on healing, and then another clear message to write.

Let faith dominate, and proceed to simply be a witness to all the miracles.

This time a flood of healing light and invisible intelligence deepened the meditative setting. *Miracles need a witness. Miracles are everywhere, and yet so many are missed . . .*

I opened my eyes, and I wrote again. Then, another message.

Courage is not the point, though courage helps. Faith is the point. Be a witness.

I think this message was about the miracles again. I could try to make sense of it but that wasn't the work needed—it was a dictation, and my role was to write it down.

Less than five minutes later another simple line.

In the prayer you know, remember, "Thy will be done" is the key.

I stayed there.

And the guide for her prayer is Mary, mother of baby Jesus.

I recognized the dreamlike flash of the symbol of a blue draped cloth. The message was about allowing Mother Mary to guide Adela in her prayers.

Guiding the prayers. How? I did not know. I was just following this session set forth by a coin from a slice of vasilopita bread. I felt it was all arranged for Adela. I wrote it all down.

And then one more message.

After prayer, there is always a blessing. Feel the blessing of holy water, and the holy water is in the body. It is the special water for the eyes.

Then the pink energy lifted. Our session wrapped up. The notes were in a list form that looked like a recipe. I shared every word exactly with Adela. She interpreted most of it for me in terms of an upcoming Greek Orthodox service dedicated to the baptism of Jesus. Most importantly, all of it made sense to her.

It was a recipe:

- Forgiveness then gratitude
- Ask for miracles
- Then be a witness to miracles
- Surrender to "Thy will be done" through prayer with Mother Mary
- Feel blessed with the holy water that is in our eyes

Adela was my last client of the day. We said goodbye, and she tucked her notes into her winter coat. It was the most uncomplicated and yet disciplined session, and I will never forget it. My task was clear; be quiet and write down the notes for this session. No urgency, and no fixing needed. I didn't even need to try to be more precise. In her case, it was all clear from the very start.

As I stepped into my car, I thought about how remarkable each client is. I wondered if I should be more of a dictation service for my clients, like I was with Adela—I simply stepped aside, wrote down the messages, and just became a witness. Adela seemed to have a wealth of support around her spiritually. I followed that support and I listened.

I called my husband to say I would be home soon. He made a quick joke that I was running "on time." I looked at the clock. I *was* running on time.

I thought about the wisdom of this Greek family's tradition. A specific recipe for a loaf of basil bread was the inspiration for Adela's session. And what a session it was! She followed her traditions when the first slice contained the baked-in coin. She would dedicate her year this way to her beliefs. I wondered about my own family's tradition: the ones that remain and the ones long lost.

I pulled out to the main road and took a left toward the highway. Sometimes I have business calls to make, sometimes I catch up on the news, sometimes I click on a podcast, sometimes I even like sports radio, but this evening I turned on a little music for the drive. A song by the Beatles played on the radio as I accelerated onto the highway.

Against the cold January air, I opened the window to clear my mind. And as I headed toward home, I thought about what recipe I wanted to prepare for my family's dinner that night.

THE GOOD MEDICINE OF TRADITIONS
Medicine Bottle #15

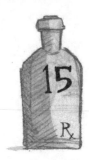

VASILOPITA

The activity of following a traditional recipe can become a sacred meditation. With rich memories, patience, as well as delicious smells and flavors, these traditions can activate a deep peace.

Imagine that you have the "cookbook" from an ancestor, a wise guide, or a holy person. What recipe are you seeking?

Meditate on the recipe with an openness and joy. Maybe it is a specific recipe from your childhood. My grandmother would make a dessert called Snow Pudding. It tasted like kindness and love and had even more to do with her kitchen, her kindness, and her sweet voice, than that amazing custard sauce she poured into my bowl.

Can you create a recipe for Joy or Peace or Love or Kindness?

What are the elements that build a tradition? Time honored? Connections? Sharing? Now fill in the rest for yourself.

My Recipe for _____

_____

_____

_____

_____

_____

_____

_____

_____

_____

_____

_____

Extra instructions:

This recipe is also your prescription for the Good Medicine of Traditions.

May cause comfort in times of transition.
Can be passed from generation to generation.

chapter 16

FORGIVE

When Pearl died, I mourned her life and the idea of never getting to learn from her again. I never thought I'd run out of time with Pearl. I had so many questions. A friend of mine once described our potential ability to communicate with deceased people, comparing it to looking at the blades of a helicopter. When the blades turn slowly, anyone can see them—but when they are at full speed, they are virtually invisible. However, if you really concentrate and follow one blade, you can see it fully— especially if the spinning slows down just a bit.

I like this metaphor for trying to understand the vibrational energy of souls. It's poetic.

When I grieve, I wonder about the survival of souls of the dead and how we can honestly communicate beyond death.

I met Amanda at a holistic health fair. I looped around from table to table browsing vendors for jewelry, music, clothes, skin care, chiropractic care, water filters, and all the other offerings you can imagine from a room full of healers. Massage and Rolfing were being offered at one table and several tables had psychics offering short readings. Every psychic's table was filled with displays except Amanda's table. I remember a simple white tablecloth, a stack of brochures, and a beautiful pendant necklace she wore over her T-shirt. She had the presence of a chieftainess. With extra cash in my pocket and in the spirit of a "fair," I asked Amanda for a reading. She is an energy healer *and* a medium.

She explained that it's all the same: It's all the powerful unseen energies that are real and loving. Then she began. She spoke to me about my parents' health and how my deceased grandparents were watching over them. She also connected on the topic of my toddler son and his future brother, who would arrive in an unusual way. At the time, I had no idea why she would say "unusual." Today, as an adoptive mom to a child who was placed when he was nine years old, I understand how right she was. She was validating, nonthreatening, respectful, and authentic.

My next session with Amanda was at her office and scheduled weeks in advance. Coincidentally, it turned out to be only three days after I learned of Pearl's passing. I had booked an appointment to see Amanda for energy healing to reduce my stress levels. I'd become entangled in conflict with a new neighbor who cut down my apple tree—one that yielded an organic harvest of fruit, and the tree itself was a gift from a dear friend. Moreover, my neighbor was unremorseful and lacked any compassion for my grief. Knowing this, I was incapable of compassionately releasing myself from my resentment toward my neighbor. I hoped Amanda could help me move through this episode with more ease than the path of anger I was headed down.

After catching her up on my neighborhood dilemma and what was holding me back, Amanda asked me about my friend Pearl. I told her what I knew; she worked with the nurses in World World II, caring for soldiers, for both enemies and allies. If she were alive, I wanted to ask her more questions about her experience with energy healing from our previous conversation at the luncheon.

"Well, maybe she is around," Amanda patted her hand to invite me to the table.

It was 9:30 in the morning when the session began. It felt like a unique indulgence for me to *receive* the care of healing. Healing is omnidirectional. It can come from anywhere. But on this day, I was in the care of Amanda. As soon as Amanda began her work, I felt a subtle sensation of spinning. I noted that it was different from uncomfortable dizziness. In fact, I didn't feel dizzy, I felt refreshingly disorientated.

I was letting go.

I felt my physical awareness of matter melt away as I dipped into a meditative place. It was early in my day and even with my eyes closed, I was both wide awake and deeply relaxed.

Emotional sensations filled my chest—I felt that anger toward my neighbor and I felt an anxiety telling me it's all much more than my neighbor. I noticed frustration, anger, more anger, and then . . . swoosh. *Where did I go?* I can only describe a sensation of something pouring out of my head—like a dam opened and a waterfall of excess flowing away.

Then, as a picture on a movie screen, I saw my house. There was a strong, steady wind blowing across our yards. I remembered dreaming this same image two nights before. It's a helpful notion—just breezing the conflict away like I had a big fan sending a healing wind across the properties.

Then a thought occurred, or was it a memory? I felt like I remembered that this breeze is actually divine protection. When I kept myself awake at night—bemoaning my lost apple tree—I'd asked for protection to create safety, boundaries, and resolution for our home. This gentle wind I was seeing clearly from my meditation was like an angel. Silently, on Amanda's table, I asked for clarity in my heart. The anger was too much for me to hold any longer. I was dedicating attention to resentment even when I knew better—knowing how damaging resentment can be.

Amanda was diligently at work around me as I became aware of the room again. I heard her gentle footsteps and felt the slight breeze of her movements.

"I just remembered something," I interrupted with a whisper.

"Mmmm," she replied neither encouraging or discouraging me.

"I forgot about forgiveness in all this living," I said.

Somewhere more than ten years back, I read the two most important ingredients for personal miracles are gratitude and forgiveness. The gratitude I remembered—not because it is easy but because gratefulness is spoken about often. In America, we even have a holiday for it in November. Practicing gratitude is graceful.

But I had not been practicing forgiveness. In fact, I was calloused, maybe in an effort to "stick up for myself," or "keep up" with pressures of midlife. I reinstated an edge to my worldview. Call it hormones, call it stress, call it midlife crisis—but I had replaced forgiveness with decisive judgments and assertive actions.

Just on the outskirts of my awareness, this remembering felt like a bit of grace itself. "Practice forgiveness, practice forgiveness" was rolling through my thoughts. I imagined a four-ton boulder impossible to move. I needed to practice lifting it. There is grace in the practice. Each effort makes me a little stronger in forgiveness. And maybe moving forward inch by inch is what matters most.

Still under Amanda's care, my list of grievances unfurled from my heart with a need to forgive everyone close to me. Further, I could see that even under this peaceful, angelic, and relaxing condition, my obstinate attitude was persisting.

My apple-tree-murdering-neighbor had brought out the *worst* in me. Resentment. I could now clearly see the worst in me. *Maybe that was even a good thing?*

After a while, Amanda asked me to sit and chat for a few minutes. She shared about forgiveness and how it is a lovely notion but, honestly, the real practice takes muscle.

I skipped past her words about forgiveness to ask hopefully, "Did you by chance get to connect with Pearl?" Amanda recalled a presence of joyful, energetic energy that showed herself youthful but surprisingly elderly in age. "Her spirit," Amanda impressed, "was so much younger compared to her chronological age at passing. I felt a spirit around me like that."

"Yes, that sounds like Pearl," I insisted.

"Well, nothing more specific than what you already know," she continued, "but I kept thinking about her care for the enemies as well as the wounded US soldiers. Talk about forgiveness," Amanda added. "There's an example for forgiveness; forgiving the ones who wounded us."

Suddenly we both lit up. And then we laughed. That epiphany about forgiveness. That was my reminder. This graceful message was inviting forgiveness back into my life. Was that Pearl's message for us? In fact, was she there all along throughout the hour? *Forgiveness matters*, was the reminder, *and don't forget to practice.* And that is just the type of message Pearl would deliver. *Keep practicing.*

THE GOOD MEDICINE OF FORGIVENESS
Medicine Bottle #16

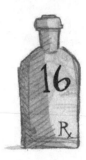

FORGIVE

The apple tree cut down on the land boundary line was a metaphor for my interpersonal challenges. Boundaries also mark the edge of our internal and external worlds. Hurt people tend to stand on the edge of their boundaries looking for any overlapping resources. If not done with love and respect, this act of edging past boundaries can inflict harm. It doesn't matter if it's with a chainsaw to a healthy apple tree, or a bomb to Pearl Harbor. Harm becomes a cycle of pain and violence.

Can forgiveness break the cycle of harm? Does it help to know how toxic non-forgiveness is? List off three situations that are ripe for your forgiveness.

1. _____

2. _____

3. _____

Commit to the gift of taking as long as you need to gather and begin to actively forgive.

This is your prescription for the Good Medicine of Forgiveness.

Expect freedom. May experience some memory loss as disturbances and grudges that dominated your daily thoughts dissipate.

chapter 17

OBSTACLES

My work to get the four-ton resentment chip off my shoulders led me to a conversation with Terry, a wise women I met at a retreat center on the Hudson River. Focusing on spiritual collaboration, the center is a commune of sorts. Terry was one of the permanent residents. She lived there year-round, except when she traveled. One weekend, after I completed an intensive healing workshop, I decided to stay an extra night to rest before the long drive home.

That evening, Terry was preparing for a trip to Africa to work on a construction project. I asked, "What's the building for?"

"It's a conference center with an *obstacle course*."

"An obstacle course?" I wondered how an obstacle course could be worth traveling across the world to visit. "For research?"

Terry told me about a small team of genocide researchers who took a census of the survivors. The project included knocking on every door around a village.

"Two researchers approached a woman who was the sole survivor of her household," Terry began. "'This woman said, 'He killed my whole family' and pointed across the field to a house, and she told the researcher that every day she woke up wishing she had died, too. 'I don't know why I'm still here. I look forward to nothing. My life is ruined.'"

"Then the researchers walked to that man's house across the field." Terry continued, "He opened the door for the census. 'I am the only one home,' he said, 'I'm the only one here. Everyone else left. I was a soldier in the war. I was violent and did a lot of harm even to my neighbors, so I always stay inside. I'm waiting for my life to end. My life is nothing.'

"The stories were extreme opposites," Terry said, "and yet the researchers noticed the description of pain was almost exactly the same. Both accept that their life is ruined."

"But the researchers conducting this survey were inspired by the truth and reconciliation techniques of post-apartheid South Africa. They wanted to rebuild this ravaged community in the same manner, by identifying the root of the pain and trauma. With careful negotiating, both neighbors agreed to meet with the researchers and participate in this project—to bring war enemies together to navigate an obstacle course built for the healing of the village.

"When they met, the woman wailed at the sight of the man." Terry was washing her hands and spoke over the sound of running water. "And this man retreated to a lone tree stump and just waited."

Terry told me that the researchers let the man and woman both know that this was a far-reaching experiment born from the utter despair of war. The course was muddy and dangerous. High walls and ropes leafed through long narrow tunnels. "None of this would be easy," Terry explained. "Only when they were ready, they could begin.

"But finally they decided to try. The man was blindfolded with his hands loosely tied, and the woman was given the task to guide her adversary safely through the course. The man stood and waited a long time until the woman agreed to commit to the challenge. Then, together, they began navigating through the first tunnel . . . together.

"While navigating climbs, crawls, and twists in the course—the victim was engaged to lead her blindfolded perpetrator in an elaborate trust exercise."

An elaborate trust exercise. I was spellbound by her story.

"The result was a spontaneous peace treaty forged from collaboration." Tears were in Terry's eyes. "And then the most incredible thing happened."

"What happened?" I asked.

"They laughed together," she answered. "And that broke the stronghold of violence. It sounds impossible. But they were able to laugh. At the end of the obstacle course, when the man took off his blindfold, she hugged him. His victim hugged him. He slaughtered her family, and yet at the completion of the obstacle course, she hugged him."

"Unbelievable," was my only reply to this story. *Not possible* was my whispered thought.

"The researchers asked them to come to breakfast the next day," Terry continued. "They both did. And the next morning, and the next, and the next.

"Together they decided to build a place where others could practice forgiveness, and bring hope for peace. When I learned about this story I knew that if I could be part of laying one brick for this project, I will know I have purpose in my life."

I began to understand why I was meant to hear this story. I was grateful to meet Terry and I knew she'd have many more teaching stories when she returned.

Terry put much more than just one brick in that building. She stayed until the building was complete. Now busloads of visitors arrive at this African center to participate in incredible acts of forgiveness and healing.

To learn more about HROC Rwanda, see their website at: healingandrebuildingourcommunities.org. According to their site, "Healing and Rebuilding Our Communities (HROC)—Rwanda strives to provide psychological support and training to Rwandan people and communities that have experienced genocide, sexual/domestic violence, and trauma of any kind; simultaneously HROC Rwanda promotes peace education to establish a future generation guided by nonviolent and harmonious values. HROC Rwanda helped to develop the HROC program in 2003 as a means to promote healing and reconciliation among communities that had experienced brutal violence and genocide. Workshops brought together ten Hutu and ten Tutsi to reestablish trust between neighbors and rebuild community relationships. HROC Rwanda currently conducts approximately 35–40 workshops per year throughout Rwanda and has recently implemented HROC workshops in schools. In 2012, HROC Rwanda purchased land in Musanze, Rwanda, to develop a HROC Center. The Center currently houses the administrators' offices and a branch of the Children's Peace Libraries and serves as a conference space to hold local workshops and trainings. HROC Rwanda hopes to add a small guesthouse on the property as a way to generate income for the center."

On their website, you can also see the bricks.

THE GOOD MEDICINE OF STRUGGLING
Medicine Bottle #17

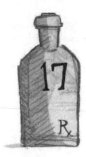

OBSTACLES

Overcoming big obstacles can bring great growth and healing. In Terry's story, she knew that the trauma of war crimes can damage whole cultures for generation after generation.

Is it possible that struggling through obstacles together, even as adversaries, can root out the deepest injustices and allow us to move forward?

If this is possible, then maybe we can look differently at every obstacle in our path as the opportunity it truly is. Living fully happens when we release old wounds—no matter what the devastating story is behind the wound.

What if we stopped avoiding obstacles and instead sought them out? You don't need to build a whole obstacle course to heal your life. Whatever you're struggling with may be the obstacle waiting to help you grow. It could be the phone call you need to make, the letter you need to send, the goal you've left behind, the overdue book, or the handshake you need to offer

Find the obstacles you've been hiding from. Be detailed as you create your own course. List three here.

1. _____

2. _____

3. _____

This map is your prescription for the Good Medicine of Struggling.

Reconciliations and resolutions may appear more frequently in your life.

chapter 18

COCKTAIL PARTY

I am listening to a deeper way. Suddenly all my ancestors are behind me.
Be still, they say. Watch and listen. You are the result of the love of
thousands.

—Linda Hogan, *poet, storyteller, Chicksaw Hall of Fame (2007)*
for her contributions to indigenous literature.

I was not expecting to have a cesarean section. A healthy mix of optimism, naiveté, and stubborn insistence convinced me that I would probably just squat in the woods to birth my baby. But, alas, it was too cold and snowy when my son was due to be born. I decided to acquiesce to my midwife's recommendation and prepare for a hospital birth. In the plan, it was going to be peaceful and easy. Plus, Cate from the birthday luncheon had assured me labor would be fun.

I was five days past my due date when the obstetrician intervened to insist on inducing my labor if natural birth did not begin in the next forty-eight hours. My body must have heard that as a warning because my water broke in the night while I was sleeping at home—a little past midnight.

When I was in my bed with contractions, at 1:35 a.m., a freight train stalled outside our window on the railroad tracks that run through our town. We checked our police scanner to hear a message from the engineer, "A temperature drop has disabled the locomotive's braking system. We are stopped." My house rumbled with the train's engine vibrating through frozen earth.

Under my midwife's instructions over the phone, I rested through the darkness between contractions. The rumbling actually felt reassuring to me in the unsettling dark midwinter night.

At about 5:30 in the morning, still dark outside, I was jolted by a loud cracking sound. Turns out, the same extreme air pressure shift that probably started my labor and likely broke the train brakes dipped the temperature so quickly that the water pipes in the basement cracked. The water truly broke.

Within fifteen minutes, the heat in the house was shutting down. Uncharacteristically, my husband asked a friend for help. Brian left a voice message for Greg, who is an expert with water and heating systems.

Before my next contraction, Greg called back to say he was coming over. It was barely even six o'clock. My heart swelled with gratitude as I remember speaking through a contraction to say, "Greg is a very, very good friend."

By nine o'clock that morning, a makeshift heater was moved into the basement to melt the pipes, but the smell of fuel was putrid and unnerving to my pregnant senses. I could not stay home. With my contractions still steady, I asked my husband to drive me to the hospital.

By then, it was a gray Saturday afternoon and snow was dusting the windshield as we made our way to the hospital.

The hospital was warm and clean and didn't smell of propane. For me, it was like a spa retreat. I paced the halls and chatted with other women walking by. The contractions began to intensify, but I was still confident that I would sail through this labor.

After a little while, the midwife checked my cervix for dilation. On a scale of one to ten inches, I was a two. I was required to start walking the halls again. In the evening, it was snowing heavily with blizzard wind conditions. I had not progressed—my cervical dilation remained at two inches.

With a windy white veil outside my window, the nurse arrived to say my sister was in the waiting room with her husband and two young children. They had driven through the storm. I was both heartened and horrified with concern for their safety. I asked the nurse to let only my sister in the birthing room because I was mostly naked except for a loosely tied hospital gown.

Taking no more than two minutes to assess the situation, my sister gave me an important message. There is something going wrong. She told me to let them do what they need to get the baby born. She was specific. Pitocin is OK, she said, she had had Pitocin. An epidural is OK, she had had an epidural with her second baby. She turned to the nurse and said she was sure the umbilical cord was wrapped around the baby's neck. Then I asked her to get home safely as the storm was getting worse, and I did not want to worry about their safety.

The midwife was happy to get my consent to begin Pitocin. I was already exhausted by the pain. An epidural was offered, and I signed another consent. Through all this, the baby's heartbeat was steady but that, I soon learned, wasn't a good thing. During uncomplicated labors, infant heartbeat rates should rise and fall around contractions. This wasn't happening. The nurses were all concerned.

Into the early hours of Sunday morning I had been laboring for over twenty-four hours and there was still no progress with my cervix. Madeline, my nurse, was the mother of four young boys. She sat by my bedside while my husband slept on a cot. She monitored the baby's heartbeat with my contractions while I enjoyed a respite from pain thanks to the epidural. The snowstorm had stranded Madeline at the hospital. She couldn't drive home, and her replacement nurse couldn't arrive for the next shift. Outside the window was a full blizzard, and the pink sky glowed behind the barrage of white flakes.

Like a coach stuck in an overtime game, Madeline prepared me for the next phase of my labor. "We need to get this baby out of you, and I'm not sleeping or resting until you're holding your baby in your arms."

Then she told me about the incredible surge I would feel when it was time to push the baby out. I remember she used the words "terrifying and overwhelming" but assured me I would persevere. She added, "because you'll have no choice."

"I know you wanted to have this baby naturally, and you are slow to progress," she coached. "It's time to get ready—you can do this."

Madeline told me to rest as she watched the baby's heartbeat, which was not responding to each contraction as a baby normally would. She suggested I change positions and rest on my right side. As I rolled over, the heart monitor made a long beeping sound that I can only describe as an alert. I turned my head toward the monitor to see the widening eyes of Madeline focused on the straight line.

I froze in position.

Madeline suggested in the calmest manner that I roll back toward her. Immediately the monitor returned to the rhythmic beat again. Madeline told me to stay exactly as I was as she left the room to find my midwife somewhere in the hallway.

It may have been five or ten minutes as I waited. I could tell by Brian's deep ocean-like breathing that he was still asleep. I was aware of a critical conundrum—my baby is in a dangerous position, and I had witnessed his heart stop on a simple tilt of my body. I reasoned the labor could be life-threatening. At the same time, I knew a cesarean section would be extremely risky, too, considering how little I moved to set the monitor off. I wasn't prepared to have the birth of my baby overrun by a surgical knife. I felt a panic emerge as no good choice revealed itself. I was physically exhausted, numb, mentally drained, and scared. With few choices left, I remembered a relaxation technique I learned in a birthing class.

I placed my hands over my eyes and counted to eight on the inhale through my nose, then exhale for eight counts through my mouth. As I thought more clearly, I prepared myself for possibly meeting my baby with brain damage from lack of blood. In an instant, my love grew stronger knowing I'd give up my life itself for this baby to be born alive. I began to feel a soldier's courage. I knew my husband would be a great dad even as a widower.

This stream of thought was suddenly interrupted by the sound of ice cubes rattling in a water glass. I took my hands off my eyes to see if someone from food services had entered. No one was there, but I still heard the sounds of ice cubes in a glass. Actually in many glasses. It sounded like a cocktail party, and I felt a jovial energy around this party. It felt as if I was present at some kind of celebration with cocktails and conversation.

Disoriented by this unexpected hallucination, I also felt a loving lightness accompanying the sensation. I am not sure I could fully describe what I heard or thought at this moment, yet somehow, I recognized this gathering as my baby's ancestors in the corner of the labor room. Specifically, about eight feet away from me to the left of the big window. I could feel the gathering as if there was a party in my room.

As I wondered what I was experiencing, a clear voice interrupted my thoughts in a cheerful but authoritative fashion.

"What do you think we did all our life?"

It was my mother's mother, my mother's father, my father's father, my father's brother, and my husband's grandfather and his great-grandfather. They had all long passed away, and they had all worked together as doctors in Worcester. These were the great-grandparents and the great uncle to my baby.

In life, this group had thrown many a cocktail party. And, of course, they would be right at home in a hospital room. It was not only the doctors in the family near my side. I sensed my godmother, my husband's dad, and my father's mother, too. I felt my baby and I, along with my sleeping husband, were surrounded by family.

The warm festive atmosphere drifted over me, and I could feel the genuine joy of surgery from this invisible crowd. All at once I was lifted from reserved dread of an impending C-section to healthy courage anticipating the adventure of it all.

· I turned my attention away and gently called to my husband to wake him.

"Hey sweetie, I need you."

"Yeah . . . what? I'm awake. What's up?" he sat up quickly.

"I think this is about to get really simple," I said laying still.

I could see he was still registering my words as he woke up.

"It's time for a C-section—I'm ready," I turn my head carefully to look him in the eyes.

"Is that what the nurses said?" he asked.

"No, but I'm going to suggest it. It's time. "

"Are you sure?" He stood up.

"Never been more certain in my life. Can you go tell the nurses?" I asked with growing urgency in my voice.

"Where is everyone?" He noticed the room was empty.

"In the hall, I think. They need me to have this baby. Tell them I think it's a good idea for me to have a C-section."

"OK, I will." He started to walk to the door.

"Oh, and wait . . ." I wanted to move toward him and reach for his arm, but I knew the risk of changing positions. "I want you to know that our baby may be harmed. He might have brain damage." I didn't have the energy to shed tears, but my heart was full of emotion. "I'm going to love him with everything in me no matter what."

"OK," he listened. He didn't know about the heart monitor ordeal, but I sensed he knew I had a reason for such a concern. "Let's just get this little guy born." And he rushed out the door. I was alone again. I knew it was the last moment I'd be alone for a long time.

In the hallway, I could hear a team of nurses gathering near my door discussing something urgent. Then my husband's voice interrupted to give them my message. Apparently, he later reported, there was a sigh of relief preceded by an immediate scurry to gather paperwork and call the obstetrician, who was trapped in by the storm at his home. The roads were covered, and I was told no airlifts were possible to Dartmouth or Boston tonight. It was the doctor and his shovel.

One nurse suggested calling a doctor from another floor. He was a cardiac surgeon. Somehow that seemed okay with me, but the labor nurses would, thankfully, not consider it. My obstetrician was shoveling himself out of his driveway as the cardiologist was ruled out.

I was prepared with another epidural and fresh intravenous drip. My husband changed into scrubs, and the nurses were joking with him wearing the blue booties over his shoes when my obstetrician hastily arrived. He expressed irritation that the nurses had not scrubbed up yet. And without any delay, he rolled my hospital bed right into the operating room by himself. He bumped into the wall in his hurried pace, but I was synchronized with his urgency. My grandparents' cocktail party gave me a strong reason to believe the surgery needed to happen soon. Why else would they break the veil so boldly for me to hear?

The operating room was brightly lit. I have never felt so naked. My legs and torso were numbed, and my arms were strapped down to the operating table. I could not move. My baby's birth had become a passive surgery. Now my job was to remain calm. The doctor cut into me with a pressure that felt like cutting through meat. I was wide awake and felt only this pressure, no pain.

Mercifully, a blue cloth divided my head and chest from the bloody happenings below. I could see a team leaning over me. As my belly was opened up something intensified. My doctor put his surgical tools down and with both hands he grabbed the baby. There was silence and there was a struggle. The nurses were concerned. I could sense it in their breathing. Or maybe even in their *not* breathing.

Most importantly, I didn't hear a baby cry.

My husband was near my head talking to me gently in an effort to keep me calm. I was sure he was not sensing a problem, like I did. I was probably very wrong about this.

Then, in a fell swoop, not unlike the scene from Lion King, the doctor lifted my baby boy as far above me as the umbilical cord would stretch.

I looked up and saw a purple, fleshy, flailing boy. I was concerned.

But my husband looked up and he saw his son saying hello. In many ways, he had a much better view. And the doctor said the baby looked healthy. My sister was correct, my baby's cord was wrapped around his neck three times, and that was why he could not move through labor. He had been stuck facing upward in my right pelvic area.

My husband stayed by my side as I could hear the nurses gathering around our baby, who was now crying fully on the examination table.

Every cell in my body wanted to jump up and reach for him, but I was still numb and strapped down.

After all those hours, my husband was relieved I was done with the ordeal and wanted a moment of relief with me.

But in a way only a new mother talks to her baby's father, I demanded as if it was excruciatingly obvious. "Go over there, he needs you!"

And in a heartbeat, Brian interrupted the nurse with a sweet, playful tone he used to talk to my belly during my pregnancy, "Hi Baby, you made it . . ."

And upon hearing the sound of his father's voice, the crying stopped, the connection was made, and finally I could breathe with relief.

To replace my husband's support by my side, my midwife sat next to me and asked how I was holding up.

"I'm fine, I'm relieved, but I'm thirsty."

"You'll be able to drink soon enough," she assured me, glancing up at the activity near my uterus. I was unaware that my internal organs were being arranged back together during the medical operation below the blue barrier. "I know this isn't what you planned," she continued, "and it didn't go the way you wanted, but you did a good job."

"No, I know this is the way it was supposed to go for me. I learned a valuable lesson."

My midwife tilted her head to perhaps digest my remark as sarcasm—I suppose she has heard it all from the mouths of laboring women.

"I think I learned compassion. I just had a client who is my age with cancer. He is scheduled for fourteen surgeries this year. As he told me this, I thought about how it was *too bad* he needed to have all those surgeries. Just a bit of bad luck. As if this was his life path and the healing choices rested with him. And the idea of fourteen surgeries would be somehow manageable. I did not get it. I did not get any of it. And now I do. That's part of all this. I needed this lesson."

The snow fell for twelve more hours that day. A skeleton staff remained at the quiet hospital. Even with a storm and a full moon, only a few babies were born that weekend. The nursing team told us they were curious but happily thankful for these low numbers.

I stayed in the hospital for six nights as the temperature plummeted in New Hampshire's winter freeze while our baby rode out a case of jaundice under the blue lights.

By Friday, we were bringing our little boy home. I insisted on classical music on the car radio as I hovered over this incredibly fragile young one.

My heart had been broken wide open, and I knew there was a piece of me now that would never repair. It would never need to.

Later, I wondered about the cocktail party and the joyful tone of that group of old friends that through this birth had become family.

Hallucination or not, it was the best coaching at the most crucial moment.

What do you think we did all our lives? They said. Words that propelled me into a state of trust and away from a path of dangerous despair. I believe all our grandparents, my father-in-law, my godmother, and my uncle at the cocktail party showed themselves to me so their celebration could continue. I'm forever grateful for the thinning of the veil that day.

THE GOOD MEDICINE OF THE ANCESTORS

Medicine Bottle #18

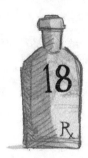

COCKTAIL PARTY

In a time of distress, challenges, and/or celebration, who would show up at your ancestral party to support you?

Who is the most likely to be there?

Who would be the most surprising to see attend?

List the three strongest messages you would receive from your ancestors.

1. _____

2. _____

3. _____

This is your prescription for the Good Medicine of the Ancestors.

May experience sudden sensations of being watched over, loved, and cared for.

chapter 19

TREE ANGELS

In the early years of motherhood, I waited with eager anticipation for my son to talk. He developed a little slowly but mostly on track for his age. I was grateful. He spoke a little later, the same way he walked a little later; as soon as my sixteen-month-old baby could stand on his own, that very same day, he walked across the room. As soon as he said his first word, which was "moon," that very same day again, he began speaking in sentences. "Let me see the moon," he said.

While I waited months for him to talk to me, he would point to light and shadows bouncing in through the windows. He would giggle while I gardened as if he was sharing a joke with the dandelions or the blooming burdock. I sensed he had started a conversation with nature. I wanted access to the world he saw through his fresh young eyes.

Down the road from our house is a brackish river that pulls up water from the Great Bay on the daily tides. The water was high on the banks as we drove past the glassy summer river.

"Wheels on Bus, Mom?" he asked. Just last week he would have said 'Eh, Eh, Eh,' until I turned the music on. But today it was worded, whole, and clear.

"Hey, before we sing, buddy, can I ask you a question?" I wanted to start a conversation.

Through the rearview mirror, I saw his eyebrows raised in what I hoped was eager curiosity. I think he understood how we were changing with communication.

"Now that we can talk to each other, I want to ask you about what you see," I continued looking at this little person so small wearing a five-point seat belt harness in his toddler seat. "Sometimes children can see stuff that adults can not. Do you see things I don't seem to see? What made you laugh in the garden yesterday? What do you point to when it seems nothing is there?" I kept the same tone as if I were asking if he wanted apple juice—playful but seriously wanting to know the mind of my child.

He looked quietly out the window. I tried asking another way.

"Some people see angels, you know, like the ones we read about? I don't see them, but do you?"

"Cheese."

Before it could begin, I lost track of our new conversation. "They look like cheese?" I tried to decipher.

"Cheese," he repeated, more assertively.

"Swiss cheese? American cheese? Cheddar, or blue cheese?" I gave in to playfulness and knew we would be singing along with the Wheels on the Bus music soon enough.

"Look! The cheese, the cheese!"

He was yelling at me for the first time with words. It was exhilarating. I turned to look at what he was pointing at. I saw a pine tree, and a poplar tree and then, another pine.

"The angels there," he said.

"The trees?"

"Yes, the cheese."

"Oh . . . you meant to say T. As in T-t-trees. You don't mean to say cheese."

"T-t-trees . . . Tree angels. Here, Mom, and here," he pointed out the window.

"Is every tree a tree angel?" I asked.

"No, dat one is," I remember the majestic oak he pointed to. "and dat one," a young birch growing on the edge of a driveway.

"Oh, so the angels are *in* the trees?" I wondered if he saw bodies with wings tucked in the branches.

"The trees *are* angels Mom. T-t-tree angels. Dat one. Dat one. Dat one." he kept pointing at various trees on our route.

"Oh . . . ohhhh! I love that I can talk with you, bud."

Truth is that in the wave of young childhood, we only found a handful of those precious conversations. Just as walking became running, his talking took him off into his own world of expression. I only had a small window that day, but we opened it together.

But I remember the tree angels, and took notes on our first conversation. Then, a year later, he got to ask *me* a question.

"Mom, is God a girl or a boy?" he asked.

I was rushing from the grocery store to the farm stand to get dinner food. Guests were arriving soon, and I was running behind.

"I'm not sure . . . what do you think?" I answered hastily.

"Both."

"Both?"

"He and she," he explained.

"I was always told that God is a 'He,' but it makes equal sense that God is a 'She.'" I found time to pause and looked at him in the eyes.

"Mom, He *and* She."

And since then, when God came up in the conversation around any-thing—holidays, death, prayers, and all sorts of God spoken moments—he'd say "He or She" and sometimes "He/She."

"I wonder if He/She can go to the hospital and help Ethan," as we drove to meet a family friend after surgery.

"I hope She or He takes good care of him," as we wept after the death of our dog.

"He/She knows!" as we listened and wondered at bedtime if the thunder in the distance would roll a storm over our house later that night.

How did I not think of this? Both, of course. Both.

THE GOOD MEDICINE OF INNER CHILD WISDOM

Medicine Bottle #19

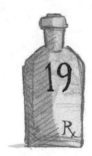

TREE ANGELS

What if we saw angels dwelling in trees? What if we had a special place in nature where you could feel a big protective presence? What if you felt watched over and loved as you walked through your home or drove down your street? What if you could remember what your first thoughts about the spirit of life were, back when you were a child?

If you could go back in time, what would be your first words spoken about how you see the world? If these words shape the way you walk through life, what would you hope them to be?

Write them down:

_____

_____

_____

_____

_____

The is your prescription for the Good Medicine of Inner Child Wisdom.

Pay attention to changes in your viewpoints. Your sight may change.
May notice the inspiring force of nature.

chapter 20

"I AM THE OCEAN"

I t was easy to know when each theater student arrived. The glass doors downstairs were heavy. The rhythm of each entry with a slam, shuffle, shuffle, shuffle, step, step, step—and then a loud sigh at the top of the eleven-stair climb. My upstairs classroom was as big as a tennis court. Then at the threshold, each child would greet me with a quiet wave or a small "hi."

When seven-year-old Harry arrived, he announced himself with an extra sigh as I noticed his guitar case that must have added toil to his trek up eleven stairs.

"Hilary (hill-ree)," His voice was filled with confidence. "I brought my guitar today, I'm gonna play it for everyone." Harry's voice was distinctive and adorable and left me smiling no matter what his words were. And Harry was always smiling back.

Every Monday afternoon my class of seven-year-olds would gather with me to create stories out of thin air and then act them out. They created tales filled with irony and adventure. They were never to be performed or published. We were developing imagination, cooperation, and creative muscles.

There were stories like the one when the turtle got lost in the woods and hid underneath a large rock, only to discover the rock was a brown bear eating a bagel. Then a bird stole the bagel and placed it at the top of a real rock that was too high for the bear to safely reach. But the bear and the turtle became friends and the bear held the turtle up as high as possible to get the bagel . . . and when the turtle stuck his neck way, way out of his shell he snagged the bagel. And the turtle and bear shared the bagel, which was delicious except . . . there was no cream cheese.

This was unfettered storytelling by real children shaped by only the rules of a beginning, a middle, and an end.

If one of the students had a leftover bagel in their lunch bag to use as a prop, that's the script that would develop. No fanfare, just ninety minutes to explore, argue, discuss, and eventually create a new story that had never been told before and may never be told again.

After a few warm-up games, it was time to start the story. Only four children were in class that day: Harry, Jay, Lucy, and Jessica.

"OK, kids," I handed the guitar case back to Harry. "Let's start the story."

As a theater teacher, I observed that children are not accustomed to the abstract mind activity of developing an idea from almost nothing. I've studied how children are born masters of mimicry, and in these technology-bombarded times, I notice kids will effortlessly soar into preexisting roles introduced via television, movies, or video games. I wanted my theater students to be the authors of whole new stories. It came as a surprise to me that children would prefer to copy ideas rather than imagine freely. An old stereotype is that adults are dull-minded compared to children who have uninhibited imagination. There may be some truth to this idea, because children *are* uninhibited, and adults *are* often unimaginative. However, I have come to believe imagination thrives with the seasoned brain. To create anything together requires authentic discipline, the texture of life experiences, along with advanced abilities to compromise—all attributes that develop and strengthen over time.

"I'm a mermaid!" Jess jumped in front of me.

"I play the guitar!" Harry hefted his guitar case up to his chest with two hands.

"I'm a mermaid, too," chimed in Lucy.

"Okay, so we have a guitar player and two mermaids," I reviewed. "But where's the beginning, middle, and end?"

"Yes, yes," said Harry. "I'll play the guitar, and the mermaids can dance."

"We don't dance," the mermaids said in unison pointing obviously to their legs that had become mythical fins.

"Good point." I was impressed.

"That's sad," Harry retorted because he expected his guitar music to be dancing music.

This was the right moment to offer a compromise.

"Maybe the guitar can play, and the mermaids can come out of the water to play for a while and get legs to dance." I hoped my idea would keep the kids building the story.

They all looked at me disapprovingly, as if I wasn't thinking clearly.

We were at a small impasse, but they together agreed to all disagree with me. Good enough.

"What are your names going to be?" I asked this in order to move the process along.

"Fredrick," Harry didn't hesitate.

"And I'm Allison," said Lucy.

"And I'm Allison," Jessica scooted up to Lucy's side as they both smiled.

Almost always I would encourage children to not copy each other—*please try another name* I'd normally suggest, but today there was an air of defiance in the room. And I welcomed it. Fact is, two names appear in real life all the time; at work and at school. Why not here?

"OK, we have Allison and Allison and Fredrick." I turned to Jay, "Now, my friend, who would you like to be in this story?"

"Uh . . . no one," Jay leaned on the wall near the windows.

"You can be anyone you want, there are no wrong answers here—we have a guitar player, a mermaid, and another mermaid. So Jay, who do you want to be?"

"I don't know," he said.

"You could be a fisherman or a swimmer or a guy playing volleyball over here . . ."

"No, I don't want to." Jay was distant and not cooperating.

"Oh! Oh, I know!" I twirled just like the kids would do. "You could be a whale! Or, or . . . a dolphin!"

Jay shook his head.

"How about a shark?"

"No." Jay was either stumped or stubborn. He shook his head again.

I decided to stop pushing. Sometimes even good willed encouragement can turn a child against creativity. Jay would get a "free pass" this week if he didn't want to be a character in the story. It's time, I thought, to skip forward.

"OK, Jay, you can assist me, you'll be the assistant director." I put one hand on his shoulder.

"Let's look at the setting then. Where are we? We need water, because the mermaids need to swim," I continued.

They all agreed. Even my new assistant Jay nodded.

"Phew, OK, we agree on water," I said, relieved. "So we need a place for the guitar player near water. Harry, do you want to be on a boat or in a field or on the beach?"

"I'm on a beach." Harry grabbed a stool near the wall and carried it to the center of the room. The beach was now underneath Harry's feet. He opened the guitar case and confidently dropped the rainbow strap over his head.

Sitting on the stool and secure with his guitar, he began to strum—not at all melodically. But he smiled and swayed like a musical master.

"Hold on, Harry," I paused him. "I like it . . . I *love* it . . . but we need to get Allison and Allison into places, too."

I was buried in the seven-year-old mindset with the students, and it seemed urgently essential to create a place where the mermaids could swim.

"OK," I stepped up and turned to my assistant. "We need to decide where on stage the ocean will be. Right beside Harry? In front of Harry? What do you think, Jay?"

I really wanted him to start participating.

"I know!" Jay raised his hand boldly just a few inches from my face.

"Yes, Jay." I was lifted with his sudden enthusiasm.

"I am the ocean."

"What?" I was sure I had heard him wrong.

"I'm the ocean!" he exclaimed.

"You mean, your character is . . . the ocean?"

Then I looked into this boy's eyes, and he looked at me with a full and confident smile. I could tell he was serious in his heart, just exactly like an artist can be when creative moments fuse with serious delight.

"Yes!" Jay declared. "I will play the ocean."

"Ah?" I was reluctant; after all, I'd already given in to the whole Allison and Allison confusion. But why was I so worried? Theater class is a place where anyone can be any character. It could be tough for Jay and even be discouraging to play the ocean. But I was more curious than anything. Moreover, at that moment, Jay was just so happy.

I leaned over, smiled back, and looked into Jay's determined eyes. "Show me how you'll be the ocean."

At that moment, Jay took the stage and just became the Ocean. He spun, and he swirled, he slashed forward and shuffled back. The Ocean swung and flailed his arms. He shouted out to us over the deafening imaginary noise of the surf. He was, in fact, a stormy sea with wild movements.

Then Harry, in his childhood genius, began to play storm music on his guitar. All at once in this big fluorescent-lit recreation room, I imagined wind, smelled the salty air, and saw the lightning crack in the distant corner where the mop leaned on a ballet barre. The mermaids laughed in abandon, just like real mermaids would laugh if they were tossed and rolled by a tempest.

I shouted to Jay as if from a rocking fishing boat, "How can we end this? How can we calm this down?"

"I can't," said Jay the Ocean as he continued his improvisation.

"I'll play calmer music to settle the waves," said Harry.

And somehow, in broken chords, Harry and Jay synchronized an event that rivaled any professional performance piece. Jay fell and rose and fell and rose. He rolled and swayed and let his feet carry him in spirals around the space revealing a clear peninsula for the beach. It was a brilliant raw interpretation of tides and waves and distant thunder until the wind settled down, and then the mermaids relaxed to a rippling waltz.

I was in transformative awe—not wanting it to end—no rushing, no narrating, and no teaching.

Then gracefully, Jay the Ocean twirled one long twirl as he descended to the floor, lying prone against the linoleum surface with his arms stretched wide. Harry gradually stopped playing, and Jay lifted his head with quiet authority and whispered, "The mermaids can swim in now."

THE GOOD MEDICINE OF OWNING YOUR ROLE

Medicine Bottle #20

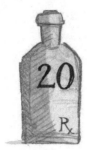

"I AM THE OCEAN"

Jay insisted on not taking on a role he didn't want to play. In this creative setting Jay took a "free pass" to watch a scene unfold from the outside looking in.

If you could get a free pass from roles you don't want to play, what would they be?

List four roles in life you would turn down.

1. _____

2. _____

3. _____

4. _____

If you found inspiration to jump into an unexpected role, like Jay becoming the Ocean, what role would you embrace and even embody? Describe the role you would choose.

_____

This is your prescription for the Good Medicine of Owning Your Role.

May experience unexpected boosts of energy with heightened creativity and confidence.

chapter 21

FOSSILS

I sat on my front steps on a sunny, late winter day. The crocuses were fresh blooms bursting purple against the season of white. The crocuses always surprise me, how early they arrive from the frozen earth. I'm never in a rush to end winter once March begins. Those long cold days are fully rooted in the possibility of warmer days, but March still holds a quiet peace that busy May and June in New England might never know.

Through the glass storm door, I heard the phone ring. It's the time of day my sister calls. At 5:15 in the afternoon she's driving home from work and that's a good time for us to catch up on the day.

"Hi Jude," I answered.

"Hey!" she replied. In one syllable I can tell by her voice she's got something good to share. "So guess who Ella requested to be the entertainment at her birthday party?" she asked.

"Uhm . . ." I could think of a bunch of funny answers. "Bozo the Clown?" I guessed, because her family has a noteworthy aversion to clowns.

"Nope," she said. "Guess again."

"I don't know. How many guesses do I have? OK, Elmo? Barney? Britney Spears?"

"It's someone you know . . .," she hinted.

"Really? Is it someone I know now, or from the past?"

Apparently, the riddle had gone on too long.

"No, it's you," she said flatly which, of course, made it even more fun because sometimes she says things this way.

"Me? What? Why? Does she want me to do pet tricks or something?" I answered with what I thought might seem like disproportionate shock . . . but I was truly surprised.

"No, she wants you to teach a healing arts class for kids. Remember how you told her you wanted to teach kids?"

Ella is a good listener.

"Oh . . . she is giving me my big break. I love it!" I laughed, remembering our conversation months before.

"Pretty much," my sister agreed, "And I'll pay you, because I was going to pay someone."

"No way."

"No way, what?"

"No way I won't let you pay me. In fact, it'll be my gift to her," I said.

"So you'll do it?"

"I'm not sure what I'm going to do, but yeah, I'd love to put something together for her birthday."

"Awesome, I've got to grab this call, love you!" she exclaimed. "And I still want to pay you!"

"Love you, too, bye!"

My feisty, lovable, big brown-eyed niece, Ella, was turning nine years old. The party would be small, with only four girls between the ages of eight and twelve. She was giving me a chance and I could barely wait for the day.

2<

In June, we began in the downstairs playroom kicking off an afternoon of activities. The five of us sat on the floor. I was prepared to playfully introduce a range of healing techniques from self-care tips to the mystical aspects of the art. I handed a new writing journal to each of the girls.

In my teaching kit, I had an essential oil collection, a yoga mat, a therapeutic table, several crystals, a box of fossils, a small bag of colorful stones, and the Book of Runes with a set of stones marked with ancient symbols.

I decided to start with yoga and practice some physical "asana" poses.

"Yoga isn't *only* about being on a mat doing exercise poses," I explained. "That is only one-eighth of the yoga experience. But this pose part, the physical practice of yoga, is called *asana*."

I explained a little bit about all the eight limbs of yoga. Too often, yoga hangs from a single limb, the physical body of postures and movements. The other seven limbs bring attention to the attributes of practicing self-restraint, quieting the mind, meditation, unifying mind and body, focus, breathwork, and observance. For children, asana with the body is a good practice. And my plan was to lead Ella and her friends through a whole set of poses that fit together to create the flowing movements of a physical routine called the Sun Salutation. The poses include fun names for the girls to remember such as Mountain Pose, Rag Doll Pose, Plank Pose, Child Pose, and Downward Dog Pose. I figured this was a good opening lesson. As I set my adult body into each posture, the girls bounced instantaneously into place.

Turns out, they already knew yoga. Quite well in fact. I was like an arthritic snail compared to their youthful version of asana yoga. Each said they learned this at school. The girls were attending all different schools, but all four girls were fluent in yoga.

It warmed my heart to witness this competency and I suggested that the group show me what else they know about yoga. They became beautifully unbound with excitement. For the next couple of minutes, I watched four young bodies float, flip, and stretch in ways I could only dream about. When Haddy, a ten-year-old, flowed into her version of Crow Pose, where the weight of her body rested on her elbows while she methodically extended her legs to float behind her, I knew my role as yoga teacher was redundant that day. These children could teach me.

For my niece's sake, however, I started to worry. What if there's nothing new to teach? Kids are smart and up to date on whatever interests them.

I decided to challenge this birthday party differently. I would go to a different limb of yoga.

"All these yoga poses were developed to bring the body to a calm resting position for deep meditation."

The girls nodded.

"Have any of you done a real mediation?" I asked. The girls looked at each other and swayed their heads. "Well, meditation is simply a way of thinking of nothing, or as I sometimes practice, not thinking at all. It is like listening to your soul," I explained as simply as possible.

The girls chuckled at this idea. It was a sweet laugh as if I had mentioned an inside joke. *Imagine! Listening to your soul?*

Emmy chimed up, "Um, how can you listen to your soul? What exactly is a soul? I've always wondered about that."

I looked at my niece, and she just beamed a proud smile as if she knew I would come up with a perfectly excellent answer.

This was a good idea for a birthday party: a healing arts workshop. At that particular moment, however, I wondered about the scope of this assignment. My heart was filled with love for Ella and also for her sweet friends. I felt unprepared for this self-inflicted question I had ignited, "What is a soul?"

I looked around for help. The garden was right outside the sliding glass doors. Inside there were family pictures behind me on the wall, and beside me was a box with my collection of fossils. *The fossils!* The fossils would be my metaphor for the soul. Souls are like fossils.

I improvised as I explained how these fossils could be like souls. They had been found by friends hiking in southeastern Canada. I encouraged the girls to take several pieces from the shoebox. The gray slate-like stones all had small ferns embedded in the surfaces.

"One hundred and fifty million years, at least," a local geologist told me when I showed him the shoebox.

"You see this rock?" I continued to the girls, "these are older than ancient . . . and once a fern grew near where these fossils were found."

"The fern grew in a rock?" the youngest girl, Emmy, asked.

"The fern was rooted in silt and soil, which all became this fossil over millions of years." I passed the biggest one around our circle. "This imprint of the fern shows that it has had millions and millions of years on earth before this moment. This single stone right here, no doubt, knows a lot."

From here I was ready to dive into the full meaning of this metaphor. I was perched to talk about our souls being resilient and lasting beyond our bodies. However, I wasn't sure how to delicately cover this topic without possibly entangling religious beliefs with bigger topics that would need more parental involvement. My mind was strategizing quickly . . . but then a hand went up. Haddy had a question and I welcomed the interruption.

"Can we ask the fossil what it knows?" Haddy asked.

"Oh, I did say it knows a lot," I laughed.

I had forgotten how expressions can sound so literal to young ears. The girls were all agreeing this was a fun idea. I wasn't so sure what the result would be, but in the spirit of this party, I said "Sure!"

We each sat cross-legged holding our fossil rocks. As I sat there, I couldn't meditate. Instead, I wondered about the next activity I would do. In a few moments, I knew the kids would discover that rocks don't talk, and I'd need to quickly move on to *The Book of Runes*. I needed to keep planning.

As the girls sat quietly holding the rocks, I was so proud of them for their sincere intention to meditate with fossils, but simultaneously, I also wondered when the pizza would arrive.

Within a few minutes, all four of them opened their eyes. Emmy took the longest to finish.

When her eyes opened, Ella blurted out to her, "So, did you get anything?"

"December!" Emmy exclaimed.

The girls all cheered and giggled. It was absurd theater. Again, I asked myself, *what have I gotten us all into?*

"What happened in December?" I asked Emmy.

"No, it's a *future* December," she sighed at me.

"What is?" Now I was starting to laugh, too.

"That's the answer the rock gave me." She held up the rock as if it had some clear writing for me to read and bobbed her whole body as a confident affirmative.

"Ah, oh, wow!" I understood. The girl had connected.

"Well, what was your question?" Olivia who was the wise elder of the group at age eleven asked Emmy, looking up from her journal.

"I asked," said Emmy, "When am I going to get a dog?"

"And the answer was December?" I concluded with a concerned tone. I didn't mean to dampen the mood, but now I was worried about the repercussions with parents. In a short time my concern went from "not challenging enough," to considering what happens when a fossil falsely promises a new dog for Emmy next December.

Part of me wanted to believe it was all possible. But I also believe that dogs and children and a family decision to get a pet isn't something a rock can tell us—even a 150 million-year-old rock.

"Did anybody else get a message from their fossil piece?" I scanned the other three.

"Well," my niece took a big exasperated breath. "I didn't really know what to ask."

"Well, that's completely OK," I smiled.

"But I know what to ask *now*," she threw her hand up in victory.

"Really," I was catching on with their youthful spirit. "What's your question then?"

"Hang on," Ella said and proceeded to close her eyes and listen to the fossil.

We all waited and watched for not much more than a minute. When she opened her eyes she turned right to Emmy.

"When you're old enough and when you're responsible enough," Ella said.

"What's that answer for?" I asked.

"I wanted Emmy to know which December she'll get her dog."

"Oh . . ." I was awed by these girls. Emmy was fascinated and resolved with this answer.

"As long as I know I'll get a dog someday." She patted Ella on the back, "thanks!"

"Someday . . . when you're ready . . . in a December," Ella affirmed with a head nod.

I was satisfied that the meditation exercise about fossils and dogs was almost complete.

"Did anyone else get any thoughts while meditating with the fossil?" I wanted to make sure everyone had a chance to share. I expected that the dog question couldn't be topped.

Then Olivia raised her hand formally as if I was a classroom teacher.

"Did you get an insight into something?" I asked as I saw her opening her journal.

"Well, sort of, but I didn't exactly know what to ask. Emmy had the *perfect* question, but I had no idea," replied Olivia.

"OK, that's OK, so what did you end up asking?"

"Well, since you said it knew a lot, I asked the fossil what it knew."

Seems logical, I thought.

I looked a little closer at Olivia. She was unflinching. And her journal was open to a page of writing.

She looked down and started to read aloud:

"I've seen mountains rise up and fall down," she read. Then added a comment to us, "I think that's because 150 million years is a really long time and . . ."

Then checked her notes again, "And the fossil said it's 'Seen the being of us.'

I could feel my heart beating.

"Us means us humans," she added, "like the very beginning when there were only plants and animals here."

Then she read again, "And it told me, 'I know the ocean really well.'"

She closed her journal.

"Wow," I uttered. I was overwhelmed. Confusion combined with goose-bumps. Maybe it was the wisdom from Olivia. Or maybe I was struck by how precisely a fossil and a child can communicate. It didn't matter. I was speechless.

I wished for another adult in the room to share an astonished look between us. But it was just me alone with the girls and we all just nodded. Until Emmy said, "I wonder if my dog is going to have spots or not . . . maybe just one spot on the back."

Olivia, now finished channeling the soul of a fossil, answered, "You know what's cool, Emmy, my cousin got a dog that was all black but had white spots on the tip of his ears. He's so cute!"

From the top of the basement stairs, my sister shouted that the pizza was ready and the girls could take a break. "Oh yeah, perfect timing," I shouted back. "I'll send them up!" But Haddy, Ella, Emmy, and Olivia were already racing to the stairs.

"Do you want a piece, too?" My sister offered.

"No, I'm good to wait down here," I hollered back up to her.

And for the next ten minutes, I stayed still and looked at those fossils in an entirely different way.

THE GOOD MEDICINE OF CREATIVE MEDITATION

Medicine Bottle #21

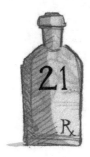

FOSSILS

Sometimes meditation can assist in directing and clearing our mind. Creative meditation is a chance to ask a question without knowing the answer.

Ask a question while holding a sacred item: a gift, a sentimental treasure, a rock, a photo.

What is the item? _____

Now, like at the birthday party, take time to meditate and listen for a message. You can even imagine what you hope the message to be. In this case it doesn't matter. It's all about creativity. Take down some notes like Olivia did.

_____

_____

_____

_____

_____

_____

This is your prescription for the Good Medicine of Creative Meditation.

May experience an awakened ability to communicate
with all things sacred to you.

chapter 22

WRINKLES

"Mom, which witch is the younger witch?" My son leaned forward from the back seat of the car.

It was just the two of us at 8:04 a.m. on Route 128 north of Boston. The potholes from this winter's snowstorms made for a bumpy ride. Spring, however, was in a full crescendo showing off tree flowers and bright dandelions bursting against the bountiful greens. I focused on driving and dreaming about more spring—the spring that happens when there isn't some place to rush to. On the stereo, we were listening to an audiobook: actress Hope Davis read *A Wrinkle In Time*. It was the part when the character Megan Murray was being hurtled into a damp, cold place in outer space. Meanwhile, our car suddenly slowed as traffic backed up for the foreseeable distance. We were going to be late for school.

"Uh," trying to answer his question from five minutes back into the story, I guessed," is it the woman with the soft voice?"

"What? No. Mom, it's either Mrs. Whose-it or Mrs. Whats-It. But which one is which?"

"I gotta admit, bud," as I slowly merged into the right lane, "I'm not listening as carefully as you are."

"Oh, I thought we were listening together. Can you pause it and go back?"

I thought we were listening together, too, yet . . .

I had been listening—but I lost track. I wasn't only hearing the story of the children looking for their father in space, I heard Madeleine L'engle's other story: the soul-searching story about life being lived in the here and the now.

"You can't feel anger and be afraid at the same time," one witch said to the children.

Then, on the audiobook, I'd heard the list of "Light" people who have already lived as humans. Megan, too busy thinking about her father, could only think of Euclid, the ancient Greek mathematician. My mind wandered further away into my own list of Light people, and that's when I stopped listening to the story.

Driving with L'Engle is not the same as my easy hours with Rick Riordan, C. S. Lewis, and Roald Dahl on this morning commute. L'Engle was challenging me. I was noticing all the grown-up messages embedded into her young adult writing. Listening to *A Wrinkle in Time* ignited my inner child's mind as I drove in heavy traffic.

In an interview L'Engle once said, "The great thing about getting older is that you don't lose all the other ages you've been."

And later she added, "I am still every age that I have been. Because I was once a child, I am always a child."

That morning I wanted to skip school and drive to the cool, empty beach with my son. I longed to stay with him and listen to the rest of *A Wrinkle in Time* with sand between our toes and watch piping plovers run back and forth from water to seagrass all day.

Turns out, we were only ten minutes late for school, which was not too bad considering the dense construction traffic. I had a wonderfully full day planned with clients and writing, and my son was looking forward to a trip to the local pond for science class.

I didn't want us to miss anything, and yet, I wanted to stop time like the book says. Or at least put a wrinkle in it. Life rushes by with all sorts of beauty to be cherished. Life is passing quicker than ever. I was thinking back to my time.

As a teenager and in my twenties, I studied as an actress and director, spending seasons in New York City, Boston, and the Berkshires. By 1999, when I was ready to forego a theater career for more steady income, I joined the dot-com boom as a communications director at a financial company. My income tripled, but my heart struggled.

In August 2001, I left that job to pursue my growing interest in the healing arts.

Ten days into unemployment while driving, also on this highway, I heard the announcement, "Due to the scale of events happening in New York this morning, we are going to switch our broadcast to ABC news."

For five brutal minutes, I listened to hospital reports of the injured and heard commentary about architectural icons destroyed. In my mind, I conceded that the Statue of Liberty was attacked—bombed probably—but it was awfully early for so many tourists to be there, and there seemed to be so many injured and killed. I switched the radio station to Boston's public radio. Still driving, I was on edge to hear what was happening. I remember the next words searing into my memory at this traumatic American moment: "The world is filled with billions and billions of good, honest people who want the love of their friends and family and who work for a peaceful life. The acts of a few who don't want this can do great harm, but we must remember, there are many more good people in this world than there are bad."

I think it was the commentary of Carl Kasell. I've searched, but I can't find any of this broadcast in the radio archives. It was the most perfect set of words I could have heard at that exact moment.

Because, at the very next moment, I got the whole news.

A month later, I was still out of a job, but I opened Magical Child Theater Arts. The name was inspired by an archetype of the human spirit that author and medical intuitive Caroline Myss defines in her 2001 book *Sacred Contracts*. According to Myss, the Magical Child is part of the human mind that sees the potential for sacred beauty in all things and embodies qualities of wisdom and courage in the face of difficult circumstances.

Myss cites Anne Frank as the embodiment of the Magical Child archetype. This part of humanity embodies a resilience born from hardship, cruelty, and oppression. I would name my program Magical Child Theater Arts, combining the lightness of the word "Magic" while also suggesting the deeper aspects of the healing and transformative aspect of the arts.

By November, I had forty students and a waiting list. There was an insatiable need for beauty and art and wisdom and courage in late 2001. Yes, I taught theater—motivations, tactics, obstacles, and objectives. I also shared my lessons on vocal training, stage combat, and physical comedy. But the truth of this program remained in the name of the program. Those magical children were rescuing me. I learned in the middle of this life that meaning does not sit waiting at some goal line. Being rich in life is being full with the wholeness on the journey. I learned that growth is not linear and rigid, but more of a collection of the experiences that brings us closer to waking the consciousness of our soul.

I have studied with healing arts teachers from around the United States, and yet it was the lessons I learned from my young acting students that opened my eyes to the sacred beauty of all things. The children in my classes are now much taller, and some are already adults. I would not recognize them if we passed each other on the street. But we were all younger once together and for brief magical moments, I was a child once again with them.

I reflect back frequently on those life-changing days with skits and acting games. Those times remind me of innate creativity and unlimited solutions. As a magical child, I learned to let go of narrow paths and allow for outcomes even better than I could imagine.

As I watched my son open the front door and run into school, I wondered if I'd been listening enough. "Which witch was the younger witch?" As far as *A Wrinkle in Time*, I still didn't answer his question, but I would begin to listen more closely, and on the ride home, we would listen together.

THE GOOD MEDICINE
OF RECLAIMED WISDOM

Medicine Bottle #22

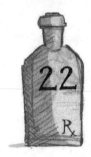

WRINKLES

Driving with Madeleine L'Engle's words playing through an audiobook, I was reminded of this author's famous quote: "We are every age we have ever been."

What ages have you been that you can recall your memories easily?

Which ages of your life are more difficult to remember or reclaim?

Create a list of aspects you want to reclaim in the age you are today.

1. _____

2. _____

3. _____

4. _____

5. _____

6. _____

This is your prescription for the Good Medicine of Reclaimed Wisdom.

May cause sudden onset of self-reverence and respect.

chapter 23

RESCUE LEAGUE

The road carved through snowbanks like the margins on this page as I slowly drove home from work on white roads. When Sage called, I had just walked in my house to gratefully greet the warm wood stove.

"Mom's not going to do chemo anymore," she said flatly. "It's not working, and it's not worth it."

My mind spun. I suddenly felt hopeless. Where was the turnabout I had been expecting? I wanted a happy plot twist. I felt devastated for both Sage and her mother Maggie.

"Is she switching to something else?" I wondered out loud on the phone.

"She's willing to do something else, but she's saying it's not worth it with the chemo. She's miserable."

I remembered stories from my godmother, who died of a similar type of cancer several years before. She described the chemotherapy treatments as "the snowballs." She would get the chemo and her body's harsh reaction would build and build like a snowball rolling in an avalanche. I witnessed this completely miserable event. Twice a month. It was exhausting and emotionally debilitating as she anticipated the next round. In this memory, I began to understand Maggie's reasons.

"I'm glad you told me. I'm planning to come down on Sunday, if that still works," I said.

"It does," she agreed. "But actually, I'm calling to get the name of your medical intuitive. Mom said I can give her a call."

I'd worked closely with a medical intuitive for almost a decade by then. "I'll email you her information, too. Let me know how it goes."

꙰

When I arrived a few days later, Maggie and Sage had a long list of recommended herbs and nutritional remedies from the medical intuitive session. Maggie's youngest son was at the stove preparing broth soup, and I noticed a big glass jar of pure blueberry juice on the kitchen table. The list was devised to help Maggie's body overcome the cancer. It was regimented with directions about what to eat, drink, and even what to meditate about. It involved clearing up spiritual and emotional issues. It centered around eating healing food, including the aromatic broth that filled her house. There was a sense of grounded support that I had not felt around Maggie since the word "terminal" was spoken back at the hospital room.

With fervor fueled by hope, I met Maggie sitting in bed reading the local newspaper. I told her to keep reading as I placed my hands at her feet. I did not want to interrupt.

"They're finally shutting down that kill shelter," Maggie folded the paper closed.

"The one down in the city?" I hoped there was only one as bad as that one.

"Yep, the neighbors complained about the pungent smell at night," Maggie confirmed.

"Why, because it's not clean?" I ask.

"From the smoke," she countered.

"What?!"

"They've been incinerating the dogs at night," Maggie showed me the article.

"Those dogs are adoptable," I said. "I've been there."

As a kid, I would visit the shelter on my walk home from school. And recently, I helped Vincent, my friend with a Rottweiler named Rusty. The dog officer took Rusty away while the dog was playing off leash in a fenced-in park.

I arrived at the park with my dog to play with Rusty. Vincent was panicking and said he would never get his dog back because another family would get him. It had not yet crossed his mind that his big young dog would be euthanized, but it crossed mine. He just wanted to get him back.

Vincent was Hispanic and lived with his girlfriend in an apartment. The shelter and police would not release his dog because he did not own a home. The landlord, however, had approved of Rusty in the lease. It all made no sense and wreaked of discrimination. So I asked Vincent if I, as a white girl, could try to claim the dog at the shelter.

At the counter, the manager was gaunt, sluggish, but friendly, until I told him I was there to collect a dog that had been taken by an officer. His face flashed with anger. I showed him Rusty's veterinary paperwork. This prison warden for innocent pets wanted to argue. I could feel nothing short of bigotry in his voice as he beamed, "I'm not sure if that dog's still here."

Knowing he was toying with me, I returned his lob, "Please don't tell me you killed Rusty!" I exclaimed. But I knew Rusty was still safe. Before I drove to the shelter, I spoke to a woman who worked in the kennel's back room. I told her I was on my way to get "my" dog, Rusty, and she said that he's not scheduled to be put down until seven o'clock that night.

But all the manager could say was, "Not sure," as his arms crossed, not even making a move to grab the leash I was providing.

"I know you kill so many animals here, it's possible you killed him already." I let myself cry and raised my voice. "You guys have a terrible reputation. You'd think you didn't have a board of directors. You'd think this was a city overrun with stray dogs that you can't reunite or relocate."

A little boy and his dad were looking at the puppies in the cages that were near the front desk. I was younger back then and I was feeling emboldened. "You sell the puppies and yet you kill the mothers," I cried out loud.

He stood behind the counter and shook his head attempting to express shame on me. It only told me more about him. I could see how Vincent was played with. It was cruel.

"You're not his sista," he frowned.

"What do you know about my family? I'm his sister, and that's my dog." I looked him in the eyes handing him the leash for the second time.

"Doubtful," he said, defiantly.

"Just get me my dog, or I'm never leaving," I stated.

"We close at four-thirty," he answered.

"Good, I'll stay all day and watch you work," I said. That actually seemed like a good idea as I thought of it. I had already measured him as a I-hate-my-life type of citizen to justify being a take-it-out-on-my-job type of manager.

Unfortunately for everyone, his job was to care for animals. We were in a standoff. It was two in the afternoon.

"Do you own his apartment?" he asked.

"I own the whole building, with my dad," I bluffed.

"Your brother said it's his dog," he seemed ready to interrogate me.

"It's my dog I share with the *whole* family." I wanted to sound like Vincent and I were from a huge family.

He just stared at me.

Suddenly I felt a clear sense that this guy wouldn't hesitate to kill Rusty. I didn't feel safe with him. He was not a reliable or reasonable person in my calculation. He looked confident that I was not about to take Rusty home.

All 5 feet and 4 inches of me leaned into the counter and now, without a tear but maybe a growl I said, "I need to go now. And I need Rusty to come with me. If I leave here without Rusty, I know you'll kill him. You guys have a reputation. You're the opposite of a rescue league, despite what your sign says. I would not trust you to rescue a goldfish."

I was not intimidated. I was infuriated. I was seeing a type of discrimination where, as a sister to a Hispanic brother who owned an apartment building, our love for Rusty was completely dismissed. I was pleading for "my" dog—the more I cared, the more he wanted to see me hurting.

"If you're his sista, you don't talk like him," he said. I did not know if this mean-spirited manager was asking me or telling me this.

"None of us talk alike," I replied, not knowing exactly what I meant, but our argument was getting much bigger than rescuing Rusty. I stayed focused.

A young couple walked in, chatting about airports and luggage. Apparently they were there to leave their Golden Retriever for kenneling for vacation.

Are they serious? Was my only thought.

The Golden was frisky and the couple seemed like they were in a rush. *My perfect moment.* I picked up the leash and held it out for my nemesis to take for a third time.

"Andrea!!" he yelled down the back hallway.

As if she had been waiting around the corner, Andrea walked out with Rusty on another leash. As I switched the leashes, I noticed the manager saw that Rusty did not greet me like I was his owner. No wagging tail. No look of recognition. I improvised through it.

"Hey buddy, why are you so sad? You OK?" I was patting Rusty's head.

Arms still crossed, the manager shook his head at me in disapproval.

I gave Rusty a treat from my pocket, and we walked out past the Golden and her family.

Good luck, I thought to the other dogs and puppies in the front office.

"Hasta luego!" I said out loud right before the door closed. I did not look back.

Fifteen minutes later, Rusty and Vincent were reunited at the park in front of his apartment. As Rusty jumped up and rolled over, celebrating his homecoming, Vincent kept telling me "thank you, thank you." And I kept saying how happy I was to help.

Rusty was happier than both of us. We averted a tragedy. Vincent now knew how close he was to losing his dog. While waiting for me, a couple of his neighboring friends told their stories about how the same incident happened to them, but their beloved dog was gone forever.

The next day I called Bruce, a man who I had known from around town. He was from an influential wealthy family that owned the local newspaper after making their money in the manufacturing industry. Bruce and his cousins inherited wealth and now are business owners, lawyers, and philanthropists. Bruce was on the board of directors at the Animal Rescue League. He took my call. I reported about the hostility from the manager. I stated my concerns about the business of running a kill shelter as the city's rescue shelter. I said he should either change their kill-at-will policies or change the name. I was calm, but I was angry.

"This is a far cry from a Rescue League that you're heading up," I explained.

I knew he did not really head up any part of this organization. He gave family money and attended board meetings. But I spoke to him like he was the decision maker he should be. His money was funding a lousy business. I witnessed cruelty, racial discrimination, and corruption that day with Rusty.

"Well, now you know," I told Bruce.

"I'll look into it," he loosely promised.

That was four years before Maggie read this news article in her bed. Bruce did not make any improvements, but the neighbors finally complained of the stench. That instigated a significant investigation that led to the reported closure.

"People are so cruel. Hil, those neighbors knew that shelter was a one-way ticket for strays. What kills me is that it wasn't until they didn't like the smell. The smell? That's what got them to take action? It wasn't all those healthy dogs who were dying unnecessarily, but the smell. People make me sick."

"I know. I know," I agreed.

Sage walked in with a glass of blueberry juice.

"Time to drink this, Mom."

"All right, Sage," she said in a tone of loving exasperation.

"Hil's gonna get me to sleep now," she handed her daughter back the empty glass.

For another forty-five minutes, Maggie and I worked peacefully. She practiced deep breaths, and mentioned that her headaches faded when she extended her inhales. Soon enough, she was asleep and I left the room.

In the kitchen, Sage and I shared some soup and then walked the dogs through her neighborhood.

On my drive home I felt hope, a relentless optimism that things were getting better. Maggie's zest was returning with her familiar desire for fairness and justice. Her home was invigorated with a focus on healthy food, helpful friends, and with a loving family motivated to overcome this terminal prognosis.

THE GOOD MEDICINE
OF AUTHENTIC COURAGE

Medicine Bottle #23

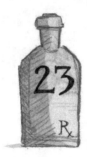

RESCUE LEAGUE

Knowing we are always striving toward safety and connection, your courage builds you and your community stronger with every resolve to live through your heart's wisdom.

Sometimes we need to be courageous. Have you ever been a rescuer or protector? Did you need to be brave? What are you willing to stand up for? Caring about something other than your own comforts is the first step toward authentic courage. Allowing your heart to lead the way tends to ignite bravery.

List three times you've been courageous:

1. _____

2. _____

3. _____

Make note of your strengths that shine in brave moments.

_____

_____

_____

This is your prescription for the Good Medicine of Authentic Courage.

Your heart may feel bigger inside your chest. May appear to be wearing a cape.

chapter 24

BRANDI

It was seven in the morning when we got an urgent call from our neighbor about their family dog. "I'm on the other side of the country. Joslyn is home alone with the boys." We could hear his distress. "Brandi fell off our bed during a seizure. Joslyn needs help. Can you go over there?"

"I'll go," I told my husband as I quickly dressed. "I want to be there." Five minutes later I was sprinting up their narrow back stairwell and I could hear Brandi, a mastiff, trying to stand up. She was on her side, panting heavily. Joslyn was comforting her.

"Brandi was sleeping soundly when she started to shake—it must have been a seizure—and then she fell off the bed."

Joslyn needed to drive her son to kindergarten, so I assured her I'd stay with Brandi.

"Here's our vet's phone number. Can you keep trying to get through? I'll bring her over as soon as I can. I'll be right back!" Joslyn ran down the stairs. I wanted to help Brandi get back on her feet. As a mastiff, she was always very strong, but now with every attempt to stand, her body was too weak and her head released back onto the floor. I called the veterinarian to report the symptoms. It was still early, but an emergency technician finally answered. I gave my best description of the symptoms and was instructed to wait for the vet to call back.

I knew Joslyn would be gone for only fifteen minutes. There was nothing to do but stay by Brandi's side until Joslyn could care for her. I waited. Brandi kept struggling. Her breath was short and labored. A high pitch in her exhales indicated she was in pain. Her helplessness scared me. I wanted to help.

After about three minutes of this type of fearful waiting, I decided to connect to Brandi with my hands. With the sensation of pins and needles, I felt loving energy pour from my hands to her body. I no longer felt helpless, and Brandi's breathing improved. Her whine of pain and panting moved away and was replaced by a deeper sleeping breath.

Suddenly, her twitching intensified. The two of us were alone together, and I prayed. Specifically, I requested assistance. I asked for help. I felt like a child; scared that this big sweet dog would seize again, scared of her pain returning, scared Joslyn wouldn't get back home in time to help Brandi.

With my hands on her ribs and her belly, I kept my eyes closed as I breathed a deep inhale and then exhaled, again and again. I wanted us to breathe together.

Brandi's head began thrusting upward as if the top of her head wanted to touch her spine. She was having another seizure. I deepened my focus on allowing healing to pour over this big gentle dog. She became calm again. I could feel her inhale and exhale deeply. I spoke gently to her and stroked her head. As she rested, I brought my hands to her big body and felt a surge of warmth. Joslyn would be back soon. I listened for her car in the driveway as I stayed with Brandi.

The phone rang from the vet's office.

"Hi, thanks for calling me back," I quickly answered. "We need to bring a dog in for emergency care." I caressed Brandi's soft short coat. "There are a few symptoms I wanted to ask you about but they have subsided."

The doctor asked routine questions about bowel activity, food habits, allergies. I told her that Joslyn can answer those questions the moment she comes back, but that we needed to get an appointment as soon as possible.

"Joslyn is my neighbor, Brandi is her dog—she will be home any minute." But as I said this, I noticed my hands didn't feel warmth any more.

"OK, can you have her call us then?" the veterinarian asked.

"Uhm, all of a sudden I think I need to ask. Is it possible that Brandi, just this very moment . . . may have . . . died?"

Gently, the vet suggested I check for a heartbeat.

"I feel a pulse," I said, "but I think it's my own heart pounding."

Then the vet asked me to look at her mouth and gums.

"Light pink," I replied.

Then the vet asked me to check her eyes. Heartbroken, I checked her eyes.

"They look glazed over."

The doctor confirmed. Brandi died peacefully while my hands were on her body. Her life force slipped away silently. I hung up and I kept my hands on her and waited for Joslyn to come home.

"She's gone," was all I could say as I heard Joslyn dashing up the stairs.

"Oh, my sweet one," Joslyn curled her body around Brandi.

"I'm so sorry," I said through tears.

"I'm so grateful," said Joslyn, "so grateful she wasn't alone."

"She was definitely not alone," was all that I could say.

THE GOOD MEDICINE OF SERENITY

Medicine Bottle #24

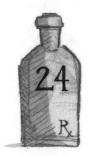

BRANDI

As I assisted with this lovable family dog, I experienced Brandi's energy field taking over in her own peaceful passing. It was an honor to be present for Brandi and to be a helpful friend to my neighbors.

Take a moment to remember a time you were in the right place at the right time to help another. Did you know what to do? What was in your control? What was *not* in your control?

What are your inner strengths that offer you serenity and clarity even in a crisis?

List three of them:

1. _____

2. _____

3. _____

This is your prescription for the Good Medicine of Serenity.

May notice calmness and ease in yourself, especially
when you're needed in difficult or challenging times.

chapter 25

SMOKE BETTER

Hannah didn't appear to be a cigarette smoker. Sometimes I can smell smoke on a client's clothing, but Hannah didn't *smell* like a cigarette smoker, either. She was wearing a navy blue sundress with an embroidered cream ribbon along the hem. She was twenty-five years old but carried a seasoned confidence with her sophisticated stride and tenor-toned voice. I knew Hannah socially before she arrived as a client. She genuinely surprised me when she asked for help to stop her addiction to cigarettes.

"Actually," Hannah said, "I have two gigantic requests."

First; she needed help with her fear of flying, because in two weeks she was going to New Zealand. And second, she said she needed to quit smoking—she didn't like the habit, and moreover, she couldn't smoke on the long plane ride.

I was a sweaty-palmed, white-knuckle type air traveler myself. The idea of helping anyone with the fear of flying was almost humorous.

As for smoking, I tried a cigarette when I was five years old after begging my babysitter for a puff from hers. We were on a family vacation, and my babysitter had taken the kids to the swimming hole for the hot afternoon. She was a chain-smoker. My begging was insistent. For good or bad, she finally let me try it. As I inhaled, my throat burned. My young brain imagined an angry dragon breathing fire into my lungs. I ran to the cold summer river and wanted to drink it. I would drink the whole river. I was crying. My babysitter was strategically apologizing with a warning that I should never, *ever*, smoke again. The lesson lasted. I never became a smoker. It was easy to turn down adolescent offers as I would never have a curiosity again.

Three minutes into Hannah's session, I recommended two highly skilled practitioners in hypnotherapy who could help. Hannah insisted that she wanted to give energy healing a chance and to connect to her own innate intelligence.

"So, how long is the flight?" I asked.

"It's like a day or more with all the stops," she rolled her eyes.

"Stops are good," I said. *That's a long time to be scared,* I thought.

"Stops *are* good," she agreed.

We laughed nervously together. We chatted about the reason for her trip.

"I'm meeting my boyfriend's family," she told me.

Can't skip that trip. We agreed again. Then I managed to admit that I'm not really qualified to give personal advice about long flights.

"I'm not a very good flyer myself. However," I added, "I'm curious how the energy work will unfold when I truly have no existing solution for you or myself. I'll take all the flying advice your energy body can offer."

Hannah laughed, but I meant it.

I decided to focus on a simple relaxation practice. I wanted to create a "happy place" for Hannah to calm her nerves during the flight. I learned about "a happy place" from my experience during childbirth classes. Hannah listened to music and counted inhales and exhales in even parts as she eased into a quiet rhythm of breath. I told her that if she could do even a bit of this during flight, it would lessen her anxiety and may keep it from escalating into panic.

"Is there a place you can remember or imagine where you feel completely relaxed?" I asked.

"The beach," she answered.

"Perfect."

As Hannah engaged in breath work, it was my turn to focus on the sensation of her fears. It makes me nervous to even think of flying. When I'm actually flying on an airplane I'm hyperaware of every sound and bump.

During a recent short flight, my husband leaned across the aisle to ask me how I was doing. All I could muster through my clenched teeth was, "promise to remind me to get a prescription drug for my next flight. I mean, a really good one," I said.

On that recent flight I tried every relaxation trick I could remember. Deep breathing, visualizing my happy place, silent chanting, television as a distraction, music, and prayers. I could say it all worked in one respect because I arrived at our destination without wearing a straitjacket. I could also say none of it worked because my anxiety was torturing me the entire flight.

"Let's just say, I wouldn't volunteer myself to help anyone get over a fear of flying to New Zealand," I admitted again to Hannah. "And yet, here we are."

I reminded myself that my work is to connect with my client's wisdom. *Not my own.* My practice is to tune in, follow, and listen. Hannah is the one going to New Zealand. My job is to relinquish any opinions or fears and simply notice what her energy body is communicating.

After a moment, I dropped my awareness into my heart intelligence. I felt some gratitude for the opportunity to safely explore this fear, and then I cleared my mind like a washed canvas.

Out of the quiet jumped in the impression. *Don't stop smoking.*

"*What?! And what does this have to do with flying?!*" said the rational inside-my-head voice.

Smoke better.

Smoke better?

Moments like these are why the worst thing I can be called is "crazy." We can argue about anything from the water bill to which exit to take into Brooklyn. But if anyone wants to escalate any tension between us, call me "crazy."

"Crazy" probably gets to me because there is more than an ounce of truth in it. I do feel crazy a lot of the time. Crazy is my gateway to freedom of thought, nonconforming, to healthy detachment, to allowing, to nonjudgment, and to listening with every cell. If I were more self-conscious and sided with rationalized norms, I'd never open my mouth. I definitely would *not* do this work.

Crazy is telling my client that the first thing her body wants to communicate around quitting this bad habit is, in fact, to "smoke better."

I was a little more than uncomfortable even speaking that out loud to Hannah in this medical building. It's practically heresy. But it was also so energetically loud I had to share it. Hannah was relaxing in her happy place, but I interrupted her.

"Hey, I just need to chime in for a moment." My hands were holding her feet. "I'm actually feeling guided to tell you to 'smoke better.'"

Eyes still closed, she responded, "That's not what I was expecting to hear."

"Neither was I," I said.

But Hannah's energy body was clear and decisive. *Don't stop smoking. Smoke better. Better quality. The toxins are dangerous. Tobacco alone is sacred. Pay attention to your thoughts when you exhale. Keep positive and send your prayers carefully on the exhale.*

I repeated the message. Of all the advice I've ever heard about quitting cigarettes, from hypnosis to the nicotine patch, never did I read an article or see a brochure that said, "keep smoking and smoke better."

Hannah just quietly said, "OK."

The session continued silently without another message for me to share. For forty minutes I followed Hannah's magnetic pull as my hands sensed warmth then cool over her chakras until it all felt calm and balanced. Intellectually, I was bothered by the disconnect of pure reason around the smoking advice. This did not fit my general medical wisdom in any way.

While Hannah rested, I told her I needed to look something up about this weird, funny message to "smoke better."

I excused myself and stepped into the corner. On my iPhone, I typed in 'smoking as sacred' in the search engine. A few entries down, buried in a Wikipedia article, I found this little gem of information:

> *"Eastern North American tribes would carry large amounts of tobacco in pouches as a readily accepted trade item and would often smoke it in pipes, either in sacred ceremonies or to seal bargains. Adults, as well as children, enjoyed the practice. It was believed that tobacco was a gift from the Creator and that the exhaled tobacco smoke was capable of carrying one's thoughts and prayers to heaven.[21]"*

And [21] was a footnote to this reference:

Gottsegen, Jack Jacob (1940). *Tobacco: A Study of Its Consumption in the United States.* Pitman Publishing Company. p. 107. Retrieved 2009-03-22.

Ha! There's something to this. I was amazed. Jack Jacob Gottsegen wrote about this in 1940. It's documented. Tobacco was smoked during Native American prayer services. Now, in contemporary times, I imagined all the unaware smokers turning thoughts to prayers just by exhaling during a smoke break on loading docks, parking lot benches, and designated areas across the world. How many ideas right now, in break rooms around the globe, were floating on tobacco smoke? And what are the contents of all these inadvertent prayers? Perhaps there is a spirit in this ritual. Perhaps there is a trace of plant spirit retained even in the chemical mix of today's commercial cigarettes.

The flute music from my stereo stopped. It was time to complete the session. Hannah and I talked about that funny piece of advice around smoking— it felt like the oddest guidance, yet authentic in its unpredictability. I read her the 1940s Gottsegen passage. We talked about tobacco as sacred and exhaling prayers.

I also noted that there weren't any insights about her upcoming flight and her accompanying anxiety from the session. I apologized. I admitted again that I may not be the best candidate for the job.

"It's OK," she reassured me. "I feel better about the flight."

"How so?" I was genuinely curious. I couldn't fathom why she felt better about flying. "Do you just feel more relaxed than before?" I wondered to her.

"Well, yes. I feel amazing—so relaxed by whatever you did with your hands and this energy stuff. But also, really . . . I just feel a better connection now," Hannah leaned back and smiled, then swung both hands outward. "I mean, I would have never, ever expected you to say that I should 'smoke better!'" She curled her finger to put quotes around the words. She kept laughing. "I know it's just not what you would have ever said to me, and somehow I feel strangely reconnected by this. I've never been more convinced that I have guidance and support nearby. I guess I don't feel alone now. And I feel like the flight is going to be OK. That's it. It's pretty cool."

Even with her epiphany, I was still stuck because I still very much wanted her to quit smoking. I blurted out some extra advice, "What about the other stuff in cigarettes? What gets mixed in? You should at least treat yourself to really quality cigarettes. I think there is some type with pictures of feathers on the package, sort of Native American looking. Maybe they're called 'Native-something'?"

"Yeah, that's a brand. I know the package but I don't remember the name." She reached into her purse to find her keys. "They're more expensive, I think."

"Well you're worth it. Or maybe just roll your own with pure tobacco. But, for now, smoke well and send good thoughts to heaven on the exhale. Actually," this idea suddenly struck me, "why don't you send up thoughts to the heavens for helping you quit altogether?"

She waved back to me as she went toward the stairs. We both shared another chuckle. And as I returned to the quiet of my empty office, I shook my head in mild disbelief.

THE GOOD MEDICINE
OF FACING YOUR VICE

Medicine Bottle #25

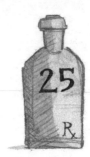

SMOKE BETTER

Let's get real about *this* topic. Do you have a vice? Do you have a bad habit that hurts your physical health? Is it a craving? Or is it an addiction?

Focus your awareness on this vice. What makes you believe it's more important than your health and well-being? List three thoughts that you may rationalize that keep you in your bad habit.

1. _____

2. _____

3. _____

Now look at your deepest needs that are unmet.

Write down at least one:

_____

What are healthier ways to feed this core need(s)? Dig into your own wisdom for three strategies to meet this need with good, healthy actions. Write them down.

1. _____

2. _____

3. _____

This is your prescription for the Good Medicine of Facing Your Vice.

This medicine will give you permission to change. Special note: others may or may not notice an improvement in your well-being. Don't expect external validation.

chapter 26

COSMOS

"I finished it." Murphy plunked Bruce Lipton's *Biology of Belief* on the small table between us.

It's written by a researcher who studied the placebo effect extensively. There is a 33 percent factor of getting the same health result from a potent drug as from a sugar pill. The placebo effect is factored into all drug studies. While placebo often refers to "fake or the trick," Lipton hypothesizes the opposite. Placebo puts a spotlight on the non-pharmaceutical aspects of thinking that something nonphysical can heal a disease and lessen pain. I'd suggested this book to Murphy. He told me he loved it and enthusiastically explained some of Lipton's ideas about how we heal the body with the mastery of the mind. Murphy, I determined, was an excellent student.

"I like the part about the cells, how cells change with thought and attitude and belief," he said.

I had studied this, too. I nodded in agreement.

"The cells are as mysterious as the cosmos—similar structures. We're all connected." He pointed straight upward. "I want to go into my cells today. I want to get right to the cancer stuff and shift it. Just like in the book—I want access to the biology of my cells."

Each session, Murphy would remind me that he wasn't afraid to die. But I *was* afraid for him to die. I hadn't known Murphy long, but already I felt close to his bright, curious spirit. His posture revealed that his childhood and his soldier training were close enough together to set a habit throughout his life. He was a man of joy, kindness, and a strong desire to inhale knowledge. Murphy was devoted to the people he loved. He wanted to live but was not afraid to die.

This spring morning was good weather for his weekly motorcycle ride from central Maine to coastal New Hampshire. Murphy reached into his rugged backpack, pulled his water bottle from his bag and took a sip. "You see, I want to get my mind and body talking so they can collaborate together."

"Yup," I nodded, taking in his instructions to me. "That sounds on point."

In last week's session, Murphy had requested to drop into communication with his cells—both the cancer cells and the healthy ones—so he could talk to them about healing.

Together, we considered that breath was the bridge to the unconscious involuntary life force overriding the body's whole mechanism. Could Murphy's cancer be battled by overriding the body's autopilot and accessing cell consciousness itself?

As we chatted about accessing cell consciousness, I noticed Murphy's wardrobe was always simple but impeccable. Today he wore a muted green cotton sweater with pants only a shade lighter than the sweater. His shirts and sweaters always followed a hue pattern: maroon/cranberry, khaki/tan, royal blue/navy. Murphy is alert to details and also pays attention to the finer points of his presentation—inside and out.

"This is a critical time," he said, "because I'm refusing the hormone therapy offered by my oncologist—that treatment damaged my heart the last time and made me constantly feel ill."

I knew Murphy was already on a powerful European drug while his naturopathic doctor was augmenting his medicine with vitamins and minerals. His medical team knew I was supporting him with energy sessions to reduce any stress in order to slow the progression of the disease.

In the spirit of the cosmos, Murphy explored the possibilities of energy medicine and unfolding belief systems to study how his body could not just slow disease but heal, too. Every week during our quiet sessions, Murphy reported to me how he experienced a movie-like picture of his cancer cells dissolving. Consistently, he describes a sensation of powerful light shining into his body. And consistently, I just keep doing my energy work to support him.

Murphy was emboldened, possibly by *The Biology of Belief*, but perhaps because of the results of a recent blood marker test.

"I want to see those markers go down," he told me. Murphy's whole cancer team, assembled across three states, wanted to see those markers go down.

When I hear about blood markers, I'm relieved that I don't hold the responsibility of his medical advisers. Instead, I hold space for healing energy around every choice. Whether Murphy chooses no treatment or chooses aggressive surgery, I hold a deep respect for his will and commitment to his own health. When it comes to his health care choices, I remain open for every possible outcome. As his energy healer, I hold a space for the possibility of "healed and cured" for Murphy. Cured from cancer. Healed by cancer.

It's one of my intentions to connect my clients to their fearless intuition. On this day, Murphy wanted to consciously meet and talk to his own cancer cells. I wanted to follow that mission.

As Murphy rested on the table and I worked to support the life force field of this brilliant buzzing energy, I used my active imagination to visualize a bridge spanning from his cells to a maze that seemed to represent the analytical mind, the thinking brain on the left side. The bridge started there and carried over to an opening that accessed the rest of all his cellular being. While I was attempting to see if his energy body would allow this "bridging," Murphy's focus was on his breath.

Just as we had acknowledged the power of breath control, Murphy wanted to access the control of the cancer cells. And with that access, he would instruct the cancer cells to fall away and exit his life. Murphy said he wanted access like he had never had before. His whole essence was searching for the gateway of that access point.

⁂

Lost in the meditation that is the hallmark of my energy work, I found myself face-to-face with what I can only describe as a protective, stern guard. This guard whispered sternly the utter ignorance of our actions of that moment. The message I felt was undeniably clear: "Murphy's request would *not* be granted." This desire for access would not fit into some bivouacked plan.

This Guard energy was undeniably interrupting my intentions to connect with Murphy's cells during a hands-on healing meditation. This Guard was something I didn't recognize as simply an imagined metaphor. This Guard was firm in the impression that Murphy's request would not be granted, the Guard would *not* relinquish control without an excellent reason—and the Guard gave me a clear sense that my *desire* to access Murphy's cell consciousness didn't even begin to qualify as a reason.

My clearest translation from this Guard's guidance was a message about the strict conditions in place to protect Murphy's cellular state. The tone seemed almost "indignant" that I'd even contacted this level of consciousness. Of course, I can only describe the symbols, translated by my words and images as best I can. But let this be said of the message I received: I wasn't getting past this Guard.

I stepped away and took a breath. I silently connected to Murphy's guidance on a level of respect to ask for more information behind the sternness. I understood this: *For very good and evolved reasons, our conscious thinking brain is not readily giving access to the controls of our heartbeat or cell replenishment or digestive process. In the same way a pregnant mother can feel love for her growing baby but not be allowed access to the internal genius of a developing body, there is no room for ego here. Whatever we know about healing and disease and belief systems doesn't qualify us to interfere with the unconscious mechanisms of the genius of the cells.*

But I wanted more. We were battling cancer. So I pushed back. Murphy wants access. This access is a matter of life, death, and at the very least, blood markers.

Silence.

Nothing.

And then one last answer. *Murphy will need to be the wisest fool.*

Foolishly and playfully, Murphy would need to let go of the need to measure, approve, or understand what his body was doing in this healing. With a mind full of measurements and logic, he would be locked out of the cell gates. The only way to get past this stern guard would be to skip, waltz, and slide far away from the left brain and into the visionary land of re-creation.

I scanned Murphy's field with my hands. Life force was balanced, and I felt an evenness among his chakras. Standing near his right shoulder, I deepened my meditation and focused again on aligning with his cell system.

As if I wore a blindfold in a cave, I slowly immersed my focus in a quiet, concentrated place of what seemed like cell consciousness. Peaceful and steady, I visualized light pouring into his body—just like sunlight at the opening of a cave.

I stayed with this for about fifteen minutes as Murphy's breathing remained full and steady. Then I began again to negotiate with the cancer cells as Murphy had asked, to get right to the cells themselves.

The room was peaceful. Occasionally I could hear a truck drive down the road. The window was opened slightly to let the new muddy air of spring circulate. We had plenty of time.

Suddenly, the peace was broken. Not by anything outward, but by this force that seemed to lock up this access to Murphy's cells. The energy was firm and unfriendly. I can barely express the surprise of this consciousness within consciousness. This was part of Murphy but not Murphy. Beyond the firmness was loving protection, too—but it was not warm and welcoming to me in particular.

I can only describe this impression as the same Guard. With a flash, I recalled that cells are mysterious, and *so* much more complicated than even the most advanced researchers can navigate. Some cancer specialists consider the cancer cells themselves are misguided parts of the immune system. I felt that type of protection.

Within the next flash, I was kicked out. I was back in the room, just standing over Murphy with my hands hovering over his third chakra, the solar plexus. I felt like I'd been sleepwalking and jolted awake.

Looking at Murphy and then checking the clock, it was time to give up for the day. I had just a little bit of time to return to his crown chakra above his head and find again that his life force was strong.

Finally, I checked in on his heart chakras above the sternum. Here I settled for just the last few minutes. I returned to the hope and steady confidence that, even though it was not today, we would get there—Murphy would make peaceful contact with his cells.

"Murphy?"

"Yep," he whispered.

"I got close, but not quite. You have a strong protector around these cells."

"I know," his eyes remained closed. "The cells are flowers. They're just like flowers."

I closed my eyes again, too. I focused on the cells as flowers. Like daisies or sunflowers facing up to the light. Suddenly, the meditative place was restored and Murphy was in a gated garden. I was in the garden, too. A garden where seeds are simply planted and watered—the rest is already there with the sun and the soil. This was access. The garden. This was the opposite of intrusion. This was where the cells would communicate to us.

We took an extra twenty minutes staying in this space where healthy growth thrives and invasive weeds are erased. We stayed only as observers, without any sharp tools, just asking to understand the cells of all healthy growth.

When it was time to complete the session, I felt the distinct presence of the Guard again, always watchful, but this time, benevolent.

Slowly and carefully I ended the session.

⅔

We continued this connection to the garden every week for most of a year. In the summertime, Murphy's weekly sessions with me became monthly. When his doctor expressed concerns about signs of bone deterioration from the medicine, Murphy decided to give his beloved motorcycle away. He surrendered to these setbacks, but persevered with all his medicine and healing work.

Each visit, we took some time in the garden and revisited any remnants of humiliation or abandonment in his emotional field. Outside, the seasons were changing and with the cold weather, travel would become treacherous. Murphy would need to consolidate his schedule. We integrated his care with his naturopathic doctor.

To save time, Murphy had the intravenous Vitamin C unit hooked up in his arm while I worked the energy medicine part of the sessions. We both agreed it was not as relaxing, but time was saved. And his time was precious.

In late December, Murphy did not come to my office for over a month. I did not see him until a sunny day in early February when we met in our parking lot.

"Murphy!" I was heading to my car when I saw him walking in the other row.

"I practically didn't recognize you," I said.

"I know, I've plumped up." He pushed a finger into the side of his face.

"You have!" I said with an unapologetic smile.

"I'm glad I get to see you here. We're in town for Helen's service."

My heart tightened. I looked away for a moment. Helen was Murphy's vitamin C intravenous buddy. They would visit for hours each week in the same treatment room with their naturopathic doctor. "I'm so sorry."

"It's OK," Murphy said. "She was ready. She was ready."

I looked back up into his eyes. "Good to see you. How's your health?"

"As a matter of fact, I'm glad I bumped into you. I meant to give you a call with the news."

This was one of those moments where I hold eye contact and just brace myself.

"So the doctors in Boston checked me out, and supposedly I'm cancer-free!"

"Supposedly?" My arms flew open.

"They said it's gone."

Now I looked away again, flashing our whole journey and holding back a rush of emotion. So many factors—the work with abandonment, humiliation, the Guard, the garden, energy healing, a potent drug imported from Germany, an advanced Boston oncology team, the Vitamin C . . . and now, this moment. Murphy was free of cancer.

"That's great, Murphy. I'm so happy for you!" The words hardly seemed adequate.

"I thought you'd want to know," he replied.

"Are you kidding? You just made my day!" I gave him a hug.

We talked about his newest grandchild and his gardening plans—we wondered if spring would arrive early this season. Then quickly, we went on with our day with cheerful goodbyes.

Murphy returned to Maine, and I didn't see him after that. Once in a while other cancer clients would call him for advice about beating cancer with the Vitamin C protocol. He always made himself available to share his knowledge and observations.

Over the years, I've been imagining Murphy still reading his books, and planting flowers that bloom for his wife's birthday, and I hoped he bought another motorcycle to ride those back mountain roads again.

Recently, yet another cancer client asked me about combining cancer meds with Vitamin C, and I decided to reconnect with Murphy to ask about his protocol and his team that got him through cancer.

It had been more than eight years since I last talked to Murphy. I decided to double-check his address and his contact information. I wanted to see if he had moved closer to his grandkids in New Hampshire—I knew that was in his plans. I searched his name seeking a new address and instead found his obituary.

Only a month earlier, Murphy had died peacefully. I had missed his memorial ceremony by only weeks and so was left, in this sad moment of discovery, to mourn alone. His obituary didn't mention his age or how he died. He requested donations in his memory to go to St. Jude's Hospital for Children.

Now Murphy was back to the dust of the cosmos. I like to remember how he pointed up toward the stars.

"We are part of the cosmos," he told me. "We never leave, we just connect in different forms through cosmic dust."

It was comforting to know Murphy was preparing even if I wasn't. Eight years after our cancer-free hug in the parking lot, in the middle of May when the azaleas bloomed brightly and sunflowers were only beginning to take root, I hope Murphy discovered with his big full heart that it was, in fact, his time.

THE GOOD MEDICINE OF BELIEFS
Medicine Bottle #26

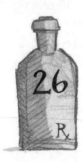

COSMOS

Murphy knew what he believed in. He needed to know because he was fighting for his life. This was his second encounter with cancer diagnosed in his body. He knew what to bring to the fight: a deep knowledge of what he believes in *and* what he doesn't believe in.

What do you believe in? Your beliefs can impact your physical and mental health.

Murphy believed in the power of the garden. Murphy believed in his sacred connection to the cosmos.

Know what you love. Know what loves you. This is part of your belief system.

Write about it:

What do you *not* believe in?

_____

What do you *truly* believe in?

_____

This is your prescription for the Good Medicine of Beliefs.

You may develop unusual strength from within.

chapter 27

SIGNS

I knew I would have a busy day. My booking schedule was packed. I was mentally preparing for each client I would have that day when I saw a very large recreational vehicle (RV) wrapped in words parked across the street from our medical building. There it was in front of the Chinese Buffet restaurant parked at an angle nobody could miss. It was a traveling billboard that had arrived overnight.

The bright red vinyl words were advertising an upcoming doomsday deadline:

Only 4 Days Left
3-2-1-The End!
Earth Will Burn on May 21
Fear the Lord and Repent Today

I looked away. My heart sank into my chest. Was I troubled by the grotesque peddling of fear? Or was my real concern, *who is the sociopath driving this vehicle?*

As I looked in the windows, I noticed the front seats were empty. In a cynical way, I actually thought: *Wow, this Chinese food must be really good. What a place for a last meal.* And it wasn't even nine o'clock in the morning. Apparently, doomsday peddlers get hungry, too.

The sight both irked and scared me. Did I feel manipulated by a Winnebago? I've been expecting the end of the world since sixth grade when Mrs. Tessman, a tough, stiff-minded teacher painfully introduced our class to the facts of contemporary war. She played a horror-filled slideshow of Hiroshima's bombing photos, while narrating comments that included, "You kids will probably have this happen to you in your lifetime." It's still a clear, snapshot memory for me. Traumatic.

After the slide show, Amy, my sixth-grade best friend, stood at our lockers whispering, "I don't want to die." I couldn't even respond to her. She had spoken what I was thinking. *I don't want to die.* A certain terror dominated my thoughts right after that lesson. Mrs. Tessman's whole class probably needed serious trauma therapy to process her great-big-certain-annihilation day. But it was the late 1970s, and we were all cognitively and emotionally abandoned to make sense of these lessons alone.

As a sixth grader, I was already a sensitive kid with a disproportionate fear of fire, tornadoes, and thunderstorms. That day, I learned human storms could be so much worse.

The big Winnebago reminded me of all this.

I shifted my thoughts to my day's first client, who would need a particular type of attention because my job was to calmly prepare her for a high-priority psychology appointment. Only eight days earlier, my client had attempted suicide. The ambulance arrived in time to prevent her death. As she arrived at our parking lot, I imagined that she would see that doomsday vehicle on the corner and get triggered to the core of her being. *Four Days Left.* That would trigger anyone. I felt a rush of anger flare back as I calculated that these peddlers of doomsday fears may be preying on people just like my client. I noticed that the eruption of my anger actually offset the nagging anxiety that started in the parking lot. Unidentified emotions, like anger, grief, and even joy, when buried, feel like anxiety to me. Sometimes that's how I need to deal with the fear mongers—I acknowledge, I get angry, and then get back to my work.

Once settled at my office, I walked to the waiting room to get Denise for her session. Her eyes looked drained, as if she had been up all night. When I welcomed her, before she even stood up, she said she was feeling low.

That damn Winnebago! I thought.

She started explaining how many issues were straining her—her boss put her on warning for lost time, her dog was sprayed by a skunk, and her boyfriend wasn't texting her back.

Maybe not the Winnebago, I conceded.

"Let's see if we can carve out a bit of serenity before you go for talk therapy," I said.

I've always known Denise talk quietly. She was raised to stay silent. That was the rule that raised her: be quiet or be punished.

I sometimes wonder if there is an energetic lump in her throat from all the tears she could not cry. As Denise spoke, I listened carefully. I wanted to clear that lump for her, but I knew only Denise can move those tears.

We talked about the events eight days before: the suicide attempt and the shame, fear, and gratefulness around that chaotic moment. Knowing she would be with her psychotherapist next, we decided to take this time to focus on energy healing to clear any blocks held in her body.

Inhaling deeply; it is a simple act, but one of the most efficient ways to restore the parasympathetic system. This is a state of living that is *not* in fighting mode and *not* in flight mode. Sitting across from each other, we inhaled and we exhaled.

The yogic art of breathing is called Pranayama. "Prana" describes life force. "Yama" is a yogic guideline to living a good life. Pranayama is the nourishment for a good life. The everyday act of breathing inhales life force and exhales spiritual debris.

Yet another translation is buried in the word Pran*ayama*. *Ayama* refers to life force expanding, enlarging, and suspending. Pranayama is known as the breathing practice that *expands* consciousness in the body through breathing.

I could, theoretically, live my whole life without once thinking about my breath. It's involuntary. Maybe when I was learning to swim there was a time I thought about breathing, but otherwise it's just what my body does naturally.

I share this all with Denise as she moves to the table and rests with her hands by her lower ribs. I ask her to be aware of her hands—rising and falling—as she inhales and exhales. Her daily habit of short breathing is so much like panting, her brain is getting the constant signal, "stay alert, crisis, stay alert, crisis."

I suggested slowing down her breath. I mentioned that even the very best lifeguards on the planet need to rest, relax, and take breaks, or they'll be too worn down to help anyone. "Vigilance is overrated," I said.

Denise began to breathe deeper. The room filled with serenity as her oceanic breathing grew stronger and stronger. She whispered that she felt tired and wanted to sleep. I encouraged her to let go and follow that sleep impulse.

I moved to her feet where an energy I can only describe as "heaviness" was drawn from her legs. As if I held an invisible vacuum beneath her feet, I sensed a magnetic pull as the thick air of tension fell away. After a few minutes, Denise's breathing transitioned into a full sleep pattern. She responded to my voice, but her body had surrendered into a serene rhythm.

I continued in my own silence.

This is when my best work can happen.

This is when life force grows and flows.

Forty minutes later, it was time to go to her next appointment. Denise thanked me and I noticed her voice was deeper and stronger.

"How are you feeling?" I asked.

"Ready to talk." She drank from her water bottle.

"Your voice sounds better," I noted.

"I feel better," she smiled for the first time. "I love this feeling."

"This feeling is what you deserve to feel every day. You deserve peace."

"I do?" she asked.

"Yes, you do, and see, you just need to breathe. Nobody else but you can do that for you."

"I'm afraid to inhale too deeply," she said.

"Why?"

"It takes up too much space in my being." Denise just paused in her path and looked me in the eyes.

"Do it anyway. Make it a habit. This is your breath. This is your life." Then I walked to the hallway with her.

"I'll try," she said as we stood at her psychotherapist's door.

"I know you will," I said.

Back at my office, I looked out the window. The doomsday wagon was still parked. This same Winnebago stayed there for a week—well past its apocalyptic deadline. I would have never imagined that a good lunch at the Chinese Buffet could save the world.

THE GOOD MEDICINE OF BREATHING THROUGH

Medicine Bottle #27

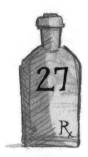

SIGNS

Do you assume that your fears are the same as everybody's fears? Not all bad activities and tragic events need to have the power to poison you or your well-being.

Which fears are advertised to you? Which signs are getting your attention and activating your anxiety?

Create an advertisement for the *opposite* of the doomsday signs. How would you express love, courage, hope, optimism, and joy on the side of your metaphoric vehicle?

Take a deep breath, and another deep breath, and now create your advertisement for well-being here:

_____

This is your prescription for the Good Medicine of Breathing Through.

Deep breathing has been shown to decrease anxiety and allow for less distractibility. May become more focused at work and at home.

chapter 28

MAGGIE'S YELLOW NOTEPAD

er dogs greeted me with a loud chorus of barks and howls as I walked up Maggie's driveway.

"Did I wake you?" I asked Maggie, who was tucked under the covers. No crossword puzzles were on her lap today.

"Oh, I wish. I can't sleep and I'm so tired. Hil, can you hand me my yellow notepad?" She reached toward her bedside table and began to prop herself to a sitting position. "I dropped my pencil—I think there's another on the dresser."

"What are you writing about?" I handed her a newly sharpened pencil.

"Just stuff that needs to happen when I'm gone," she said.

"Like a will?" I asked.

"Exactly like a will."

"That's probably smart to do, just in case . . ."

"It's not just in case, Hil," she interrupted. "I am dying, and I want to make sure everything is clear."

I was not ready to process what Maggie wanted me to know. From my perspective, she had so much energy and focus. Even as her body seemed tired, Maggie was such a force of life. I silently struggled. Her resolve and her acceptance of death was difficult for me. I sat down on the edge of her bed and just listened.

Maggie told me she was writing instructions for the house. I watched her scribble the name of the plumbing company who would need to fix the hot water tap in the bathroom.

"Oh, so you'll finally have a hot shower after you're not here anymore?" I tried to make a light joke.

"I don't mind the cold."

"Really?" I doubted.

We started to talk about her dog Duncan, the exact treats he liked, his feeding schedule, and how to groom his thick coat. Suddenly, the phone on the bedside table rang. I reached over and handed her the corded receiver.

"Hello," she answered softly.

"Hey Mom, it's Matthew."

"I know, hello Matthew," she sighed.

"How are you doing, Mom?"

"Not well," Maggie replied.

"I want to talk to you." I overheard his voice as if he were in the room with us.

"Go ahead," she said blandly to him. I stood to go to the kitchen, check on the dogs, grab a glass of water . . . all I could do to give them privacy.

As I walked away I heard Matthew say, "I've been talking to my therapist and I want to share some thoughts with you. There's so much, Mom, just so much."

I got the dogs ready for a walk, because this was bound to be a long phone conversation. As I reached for the leashes, I heard Maggie's voice raise.

"I don't have time for this Matthew. I feel lousy, and I'm dying. I'm sorry but I'm not interested, and this is not the time." I heard the receiver hang up with a clunk.

"Everything OK?" I leaned in her doorway.

"Yes," she waved me in. "Please, come back. I wish I didn't answer that call."

I put a glass of water on the table next to the phone. Maggie put her notebook down.

"I'm just so tired, Hil."

"I know." I sighed. I knew she was tired. Tired of her disease. Tired of her struggle. And tired from this last call with her son Matthew, although I would never learn exactly why. I did know that she was doing her best, and maybe so was Matthew.

Without any more words, we began another energy healing session. Maggie began to drift off to sleep as I focused on a cold cavity of space floating right above her navel area.

"I'm not afraid to die," she whispered. "I'm just afraid to see my mother in heaven. I don't want to see her ever again."

"I think you'll feel better when you get to sleep. Just rest," I said as my thoughts began to wonder about the stories I would never know.

I brought my hands to her feet, connecting her whole body with an energy flowing through my hands that was both cleansing and embracing, as if a boost of healing light appeared to fill the cavity.

"That feels good," she said.

"I'm never sure," I said as I wondered if I was really helping at all.

"Hey Hil, you're very good at this . . ."

"Not good enough." I should not have said this. My self-doubt was crossing a boundary, but I was feeling defeated.

Maggie reached for my arm.

"Hil, you've taken my pain away when nothing else worked. And you can get me to sleep, which is a gift like no other. You are very good at this. You should keep doing this your whole life."

"I'd like to," I said.

"Good." She let go of my arm and closed her eyes again. "You should."

A few moments later, Maggie fell asleep.

THE GOOD MEDICINE OF YOUR LIFE NOTES
Medicine Bottle #28

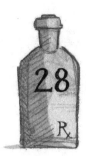

MAGGIE'S YELLOW NOTEPAD

Maggie was often writing notes when I visited. She could be scribbling a list or doodling an idea. There were pads of pages filled with journal entries. As she prepared for her death, she took one page and wrote instructions about what mattered most.

Here it is. This page. Your page to make all the notes for someday when your loved ones will get to read about all that matters to you. What do you want to say? What truths do you need to tell?

Just like Maggie, fill this page:

_____

_____

_____

_____

_____

_____

_____

This is your prescription for the Good Medicine of Your Life Notes.

Your days are filled with the purpose you describe above.

chapter 29

HERON

Randall is a fit and healthy man in middle age. He returns monthly for sessions requesting balance and insight around his health and his lifestyle.

Sometimes my work is to simply translate the messages that arrive during the energy balancing. In one crucial session, as I focused on energy healing near his right knee, a clear image of a blue heron flashed into my thoughts.

The heron is a power animal that fits perfectly with the guidance Randall needed. The heron is such a pristine and independent spirit—it calls us to delve deeper in order to know ourselves. Perfect for my client who was at a time in his life where he needed to discover a new path as his children moved away and his marriage struggled. Heron would connect him.

According to North American Native tradition, the Blue Heron is a symbol for self-reflection. In *Medicine Cards*, a book by Jamie Sams and David Carson, Blue Heron is depicted in this poem:

Thank you sacred Waterbird
For sending reflections to me
The mirrors of the quest for life
The worlds that live inside me.

But I had an obstacle to overcome. I had a memory that involved this type of bird related to a disturbing event about ten years earlier. I felt unusually agitated. I have a not-so-light association with herons, and in the middle of Randall's session, my stomach tightened, and my intuition stalled.

I was wrapped up thinking about a day many years ago, on a sunny spring afternoon, watching a blue heron being harassed by a mean-spirited teenage boy.

I remembered the small outboard motor pitching a high growl amplified over the otherwise quiet lake water. What made the sound unbearable was the repeated rise and fall of the engine. Growl, whine, putter, silence . . . growl, whine, putter, silence . . . breaking for less than a minute then repeating over and over. From the inside of the small cabin where I worked, it was the silent break that became most annoying, offering a false hope that the boat was gone until the inevitable rise of the outboard sound again.

On that calm spring weekday, the lake was gradually blossoming after months of snow and ice. Knowing rapidly approaching hot days would make these quiet days on this lake a rarity, the gaps of silence that afternoon were even more fragile.

Finally, with an annoyed lurch, I pulled open the glass sliding door and stepped fully into the view of the lake. It was calm, but I knew now to just wait a moment. I was scouring for some motorized watercraft. Instead, I was drawn in by an elegant gray bird coasting over the ripples. A common but always magnificent sighting—the Great Blue Heron stretched its sleek neck forward lifted by the grand gray wings. The long legs seemingly rested in the air until this bird landed precisely beside a young weeping willow tree.

Suddenly I was jolted, although I had been expecting it, by the growl reared from my far left. A small metal Boston Whaler craft cut across the lake in the heron's path. The boat stopped twenty feet from the bird, then puttered as close as an outboard engine can come to the shore without scraping on rocks.

In the boat was a lone teenage boy—I guessed he was fifteen years old. He cut the engine. Silence again. Then he reached for something on the floor. To my horror, I saw it was a slingshot. A big, orange Y-shaped apparatus. He aimed it toward the bird, fired his shot, and the bird lifted again in flight—soaring toward another spot on the shore. And still, again the engine revved up . . . growl, whine, putter . . . and he chased the bird, then shot at it again. This went on for an hour.

I wanted to get in my own boat and approach this boy to tell him, "For God's sake, leave the bird alone." But my boat was a canoe with just one paddle. I was afraid of my own rage to confront him. I wanted to ask him where he got the idea he could torment and threaten injury on this innocent member of our natural neighborhood.

But I didn't get in the canoe. I stayed on shore.

I felt helpless and infuriated at the same time. As I procrastinated and fretted, after an hour, the heron eventually flew beyond the reach of the slingshot and the boy retreated. I figured the boy invariably returned to his home to begin his next sadistic task. I hated that motorboat boy. He and his little boat represented almost everything wrong with humanity as I judged it: loud, invasive, disrespectful, and oblivious to disturbing nature.

When I think of Blue Heron, this story sits somewhere in the files of other impressions this magnificent power animal: Sage's gorgeous tattoo of a heron, my walks with my baby in the stroller with frequent sightings of a heron, and of course, the written records of Native American teachings about animals providing messages of wisdom and protection.

But with Randall, it was this harsh Blue Heron and slingshot memory that, uncharacteristically for me, crashed through my concentration. I knew I needed to push past these negative associations. Blue Heron medicine is a blessing, and my client has a strong connection to this medicine. I needed to get out of the way.

During his session, it became clear that it was time to clear *my* toxic memory. And as I accepted that notion, it also became clear that Blue Heron medicine had arrived as a symbol for torment and vulnerability for both of us.

In the tranquil setting of my office, with my client relaxed while an unseasonable rainstorm drummed outside the windows, I asked silently for a more in-depth understanding. *Why do I remember this story so strongly now? Why had it prevailed in my connection to this power animal today? How is this helping Randall today?* It was time for me to let go of my old shame of humanity and anger at the teenager from that day. *Letting this go is not going to be easy.*

I took a deep breath and bowed my head to pull my thoughts away from my client's energy field. I took on the perspective of the bird. I felt strong wings. Very strong. In another flash, I became aware that the heron could have flown far beyond the boy's reach on the first flight. Engaging in the chase was a choice for the heron. *Maybe even a game.* This bird could have flown higher or farther—the heron was not trapped at all. And yet, I always assumed that the bird was completely trapped. That was the story I told myself.

I understood the freedom now, but this memory of the teenage boy still brought, I had to admit, a terrible feeling of hate to my heart. It was the *all-that-is-wrong-with-humanity* sort of hate. One truth I have learned to embrace is that hate, anger, and worry cannot coexist with intuitive energy healing. That requires love. So I went to that boy's perspective. Today he would be in his thirties. The boy from that day was gone. I took some comfort in that.

I was standing on the right side of my client, near his upper torso, when it suddenly became clear that just as the bird could have flown farther and higher, this slingshot boy could have aimed closer and tried harder to inflict injury. In an instant I felt an understanding that *the boy was longing to keep the bird in flight*. Like me, he was awed by the spectacle of the wingspan—only, like a boy with a boat, he got closer.

As Jamie Sams and David Carson write:

Heron flies over those who are unaware of who they are and where they belong in this world. Gently dropping a blue feather to them, Heron asks that they follow intuition and begin the empowering journey towards self-realization.

But I did not yet have these words to reference while I was with my client; the *Medicine Card* book was on my shelf at home. Within the healing session of Randall's energy work, I experienced a lifting of personal shame—the type that lingers with hate. I was ready to realign with a much different picture.

I was released from my own trappings of my story filled with fear and judgment. I could focus more clearly on my client now. The energy healing would work with both of us now, because Heron's blue feather had landed on me, too.

THE GOOD MEDICINE OF STRONG GUIDANCE

Medicine Bottle #29

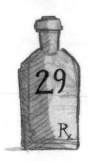

HERON

With the blue feather lesson, I realized the heron could simply set its own course and fly away. If you have been bouncing back and forth being chased by a metaphorical slingshot, think about setting a new path. What type of quiet guidance would help you find a new flight pattern?

Listen for insights and moments of reflection as your old paths and your new paths collide. What new direction will you go to? Were you just playing a game? Chart a new course that sets you free from the back and forth. Draw a map away from the slingshots in your life. Don't forget that life can be more playful than we once believed.

Use this space below, or use a separate sheet of paper:

This map is your prescription for the Good Medicine of Strong Guidance.

You may discover new territories and hidden treasures are even closer than they appeared to be.

chapter 30

LAST WISHES

The routines after death can be oddly comforting, predictable, and invisible. In most deaths I've experienced, a professional undertaker will handle the details of the deceased body. A clean, swift, and sterile service in exchange for a tactfully delivered invoice. But all this leaves almost no room for adventure.

I wouldn't say Maggie was cheap in terms of budgeting but, more like, wisely frugal. She spent very little money, kept an uncluttered house, worked a good real estate job, and sold goods at a flea market on the weekends. She saw no need for lavish expenditures at her death—she told us she figured she'd be dead anyway. And above all, what does a professional undertaker have that the direct-death-van-pickup-team doesn't have? My answer now from the living person's perspective . . . a great deal.

In her careful planning and preparation, Maggie announced that she did not want to pay an undertaker to care for her body. She considered it an unnecessary expense. She researched and found a more efficient way to arrange her body's removal. Up beyond Massachusetts' border, there's a wholesale crematory in New Hampshire that will pick up a dead person, skip the coffin part, cremate, and return the ashes in a small cardboard box.

I was home in the morning when I got the call. It was Sage, simply saying, "She's gone."

She described that it was peaceful and that Maggie died in the briefest moment. The hospice nurse stepped out of the bedroom with Sage to fetch some tea in the kitchen. On this day, her passing was expected. The nurse said this was the best type of passing Maggie could have ever wanted.

Before I hung up, I asked, "Is anybody coming to help you with her body?"

"Um, soon," Sage recalled. "The nurse called the company. They're on their way from New Hampshire. I'm alone now."

I would also be on *my* way from New Hampshire. I wanted to leave right away, but I was torn because I did not want to see Maggie's dead body.

I decided to get in my car. As I started the ignition, I felt heartbroken. Maggie surrendered to the cycle of life much more gracefully than I was ready to accept her death.

Devastated, I wanted to see Sage as soon as possible. But I wanted to remember Maggie's spirit, her laugh, and our last conversations. I wanted to remember her alive. I guess I wanted to avoid the shock of seeing Maggie without her bright life force.

I stopped at my local favorite health food store to gather a supply of vegan comfort food to keep my friend fed during her grief. Soups, muffins, tabbouleh, even a sweet carrot cake. Then I took the back roads instead of the straight line of the interstate highway. I needed the comfort of a beautiful scenic route. The big highways would be too frenetic. These roads would add a few miles to the trip, but a few extra minutes may assure there would be no chance of bumping into Maggie's body before it was removed from the house.

As I entered Maggie's neighborhood, there were construction vehicles installing massive new sewage pipes right in front of her home. Also, directly across the street, three men were loudly roofing with nail guns while blaring heavy metal tunes from an old boom box. Banging, clanging, squealing of construction wheels, and AC/DC's "Highway to Hell" on a static-filled station. I am not kidding. This was the song blaring when I arrived. It was the opposite of peace. *No wonder Maggie chose that early morning to die. It was a good time to leave.*

Perched on a parked sewage pipe was my friend Sage. My heart dropped; she was waiting outside for me. I had taken too long. I jumped out of the car calling to her, "I'm sorry! I have food! How are you holding up?"

"I'm fine," she smiled. "I'm just looking for the van. It's either running late or lost. I have been trying to reach the pickup guy—his office says he'll be here soon."

Sage was over two hours from losing her mom, all alone, and entangled in this odd scenario. She said she was sitting outside on the concrete pipe because she didn't want to be alone in the house with her dead mother. As friends, we reflected on this bizarre predicament—both admitting it was a little funny-ironic that Maggie's cost-saving wishes she had so earnestly directed weren't going so smoothly. I climbed up on the sewage pipe to join Sage. We shared a muted chuckle and waited together.

It could have been worse than waiting for a van. This was actually a compromise for Maggie. Her *real* final request was to be thrown in the back of her Ford Escort station wagon and driven up to the wholesale crematorium by Sage. But that plan, we all learned only a week before Maggie passed, was illegal. You can not transport a dead body over state lines for more reasons than I want to list.

Actually, the dead-body-pickup van never arrived that morning. But the driver, a guy I will never forget, named Rudy, did. He walked up the road like a knight out of battle. His speakerphone clipped to his hip broadcasted loudly all the other stops he was running very late for. Pointedly, these were the stops to pick up *other* dead bodies. Rudy introduced himself while ignoring the loudspeaker announcing addresses from his hip. Oddly, I found comfort in the dispatcher's voice, knowing people were dying everywhere. This van accident was creating a really bad "day at the office," Rudy told us.

Apparently, Rudy drove the company van right into a construction hole that popped a tire and ripped the front axle. It was parked only a few blocks away but not drivable. Now, a tow truck was on the way. So close. But so far. He casually informed us that we'll need to wait for the backup van, which was over an hour away.

It brought no comfort when Rudy assured us that this delay in removal would not become a health hazard for nine more hours. That's when Maggie's body would be dead for twelve hours total. He described in detail what would happen to the body over the next few hours—the smells, the rigor mortis— and about the health laws regarding dead bodies. I looked at my friend to offer some support or distraction—but she didn't seem to hear his words. Mercifully, shock protected her.

A car arrived at a passing speed but quickly swerved up the driveway to park at the house. It was Beth. Her thick red hair was collected on top of her head. I imagined she was rolling up her sleeves as she shouted up to us on the sewage pipes, "What are you doing outside? Is she in there?" Pointing to the house, "I'm going in."

Fearless, I thought.

We jumped down from the sewage pipes to meet her. And just like that, we followed our mighty leader, Beth, into the house.

Rudy followed, too. We didn't even introduce him to Beth. He talked and we walked. He talked about more dead bodies, bad days on the job, his angry boss, the trouble he's going to be in for damaging the company van-hearse, unusual death stories, and way too many details. If there was ever an opportunity to accuse a person of providing too much information, Rudy was not just an offender, he was a champion at it. On a scale of one to ten, he would rate at eleven.

Actually, Rudy had many, many "champion" moments. Time had passed with Rudy's stories and we noticed the replacement van was now very late. After waiting almost two more hours, in polite desperation, we all agreed that Rudy should stand outside to direct the van driver past the construction obstacles in order to access the driveway. This bizarre scenario was quickly devolving into a pulp fiction plot. Rudy agreed to direct traffic and exited the house.

It was quiet. Painfully quiet. I missed him. I missed Rudy's loud and aggressive voice. I couldn't believe it.

Because the open bedroom was only a step away, across from the bathroom, which I desperately needed to use, I would have to see Maggie's body. When fear could not hold me back any longer, I conjured a burst of courage as I walked over to her room. I saw a gray, thin, still body. Her expression was calm. Was she almost smiling?

I looked at Maggie's dead body and it was okay. I felt more courage surge through me, the courage that appears especially when facing a dreaded fear. Seeing Maggie's body unlocked something in my heart. I felt profound relief. I could think more clearly in that moment. I could focus on what Maggie wanted and what Sage needed. Now the van just needed to arrive. I hopped into the bathroom, and when I walked out I thought about what was clearly our next step: writing her obituary.

But the van didn't arrive. Rudy came back to the house with his squawking speakerphone as he explained that the pickup van got to the neighborhood to find the construction crew blocking the road. The new driver, not privy to the urgency of this matter, left to find a place to buy lunch, take his break, and called Rudy to apologize for this little delay.

Without asking another question, I threw on my shoes and ran down the driveway to tell the construction group, seven men in yellow helmets, to *please* let the white van through to pick up the dead body in this house. I admit it was satisfying to silence this boisterous group of workers with such a pure, practical, and honest statement, "We have a dead body here."

The outdoor air inspired me. When I returned inside it was apparent that it was time to address Maggie's body in a sacred manner. This mile-long gap between the kitchen table and the deathbed needed to be closed. This was not a sitcom nor pulp fiction—it was time to engage in this reality of preparing her body for departure.

Why had I been so reluctant to be with Maggie after her death? We had been together throughout her fight with cancer. I traveled to her bedside for months. I was humbled to learn my job was to assist her toward a peaceful death. Maggie and I talked about death—we cried together, we laughed together—and at one distinct shared moment, I even felt a little envious of her because I sensed she was embarking on an exquisite journey to the great beyond. Why then, would I not take this one last moment to honor her?

So when Rudy went back outside to wait in the driveway, the three of us, women in our thirties, stood around her body. Spontaneously, we found ourselves in a ritual. While Beth burned sage, I placed clear crystals and colorful stones of blue, orange, green, white, purple, and red around her head and torso. It seemed like a symbol of closure. I wanted to circle Maggie's body because it reminded me of stories I had heard about burying queens in more ancient times. We were all three following our instincts to honor and prepare Maggie's body.

I recited a Prayer of Protection:

The Light of the Universe Surrounds Us
The Love of the Universe Enfolds Us
The Power of the Universe Protects Us
The Presence of the Universe Watches Over Us
We Are Surrounded and Protected by Love

I noticed with my right hand that the subtle energy field around Maggie's head was still vibrating. Could I say it even felt active? I placed my hand on top of her head, the seventh chakra area, to open a connection of spiritual consciousness. I felt a full, warm, airy sensation float up and above her eyes. Then, almost immediately, her head was in a calm, silent, cloudy heaviness consistent with the rest of her whole dead body. It no longer felt alive.

As Beth and I cared for Maggie, Sage wept at her feet, and we all acknowl-edged that we were exactly where we were supposed to be. My friend, her friend, her mother, and me were together. All four of us, stripped of conve-niences and cushions, had found our way back to some kind of goodbye ritual. It felt familiar. It was intuitive. It was as if we simply remembered how to prepare Maggie for departure.

Our ritual was broken when the dogs barked at the new van as it methodi-cally backed into the driveway. *Beep, beep, beep.* Two men arrived and Maggie's body was unceremoniously bagged and strapped to a metal support system. They carried her down the narrow stairs, banging into the walls. Rudy yelled instructions to his team like they were moving a couch. We held the dogs back.

"Watch that corner," shouted Rudy. "We're gonna hafta tilt it back here . . . hold the second door there . . . got it? OK? OK."

The van doors slammed. Sage signed papers on a clipboard. And that was it. Gone. I am so grateful we took time to say goodbye.

The day was far from over, but the worst had passed. We wrote the obit-uary and removed the mattress. With her empty bedroom, I discovered the most authentic proof of life force energy: the void that appears when a person is removed in a body bag. The void is tangible.

Just when I began to feel myself unwinding into grief, Sage picked up the yellow notepad and read, "Hilary will lead my celebration service at the house."

When Maggie could have counted her days on one hand, and her belong-ings became only a bed, a nightgown, a pencil, and a writing pad, she still kept organizing us. I reluctantly felt the terrific honor of responsibility with her instruction.

I thought *No, please, really? What?* I was surprised. *How can I manage this?* This felt far outside my competency. Also I despaired, *what about me?* I needed to mourn. I had no idea how to do this and I did not feel strong enough to find ideas. I thought of arguing about the notepad—that her death might make this written request irrelevant now. *Does her dying instruction still hold? Can I say no?* After all, she's not here to uphold it.

But I soon came to accept, that's not how deathbed requests work. Instead, these words were gilded in the minds and hearts of her family as doctrine.

Torn within my commitment, I still wanted "out." *Why can't I put on a black dress and just show up quietly,* I begged to myself, *to listen obediently to someone else conducting this ceremony—a priest, a rabbi, or a minister—anybody more trained in this art of leading funerals?*

Finally, I resolved that I had no choice in the matter. When it's a dying wish, I decided, it stands as orders. So I began to plan.

I started to explore and research the topic of death ceremonies from the computer. What is a funeral, a memorial, or a celebration of life service anyway? Turns out, across humanity we all share in common these unifying elements to honor the dead. It doesn't matter what tradition we hail from. Built into our deepest habits, culture by culture, is a shared pattern of behavior to heal through the death of a loved one.

- Gather together.
- Collect this deceased one's soul through memories shared.
- In prayer, or a moment of silence, we send all pieces of the soul back to the one we are gathered for.
- Feel the loss anew. The veil of shock begins to dissolve. The reality of life without this soul's physical body begins to take hold.
- Support each other, for we are the ones left behind.
- Send blessings and goodwill to each other as we return to our separate lives.

This plot was outlined. Now I needed time to prepare for the celebration. That night, I drove through the dark to sleep in my own bed.

THE GOOD MEDICINE OF BREAKDOWNS
Medicine Bottle #30

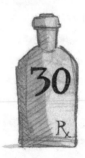

LAST WISHES

Shortcuts. Broken rules. Breakdowns. Surprises. These are all potential invitations for adventures in growth. It is only through adventure that we discover our true strengths.

Think of *one* time when you experienced an unexpected adventure. (You have had plenty!) Write it down.

_____

Now list your unexpected strengths revealed in this unexpected adventure.

1. _____

2. _____

3. _____

This is your prescription for the Good Medicine of Breakdowns.

May discover a respectful love for yourself and a trust in your future,
no matter what happens.

chapter 31

DENVER ANGELS

Across the aisle, my eight-year-old son pushed himself up to see out the window on his first journey into the sky. Leaning across the seats, he asked if I wanted to see out the window, too. I smiled and quickly replied, "No thanks." I tried to be composed. My son couldn't see my sweaty palms. I didn't want him to wonder about any fears. It was his first flight. I was excited about this family trip. My husband and I were taking him with us to Florida for vacation.

I knew I was safe in the air and simply wanted to find peace for the flight. More importantly, I wanted to be a good role model for my son and not allow my fears to control me. But even with all I've learned in my sessions, I was still physically unnerved while flying. I knew better. Now I wanted to feel better.

With a few more hours to endure on our flight, I recalled my session with Vanessa, another client who also had a fear of flying. Her primary care physician gave her prescription medication for her in-flight anxiety with a recommendation to book a session with me to alleviate any stress before the trip.

Truth is, before I see each and any new client, I get a little bit nervous. It surprises me, but the nerves are undeniable. There isn't much I can do to prepare for whatever my client's needs may be. To do my work with integrity means I defer to the unpredictability of the process.

I've learned this by experience. Especially the first time I meet a client. For example: I've been asked to help with fainting spells and was quickly uncovering trauma from an unreported rape. Another time, I was directed to assist in the healing of a digestive tract disorder to reveal it was related to an unresolved blunt force injury. I've had four clients within a year all with chronic joint pain that had healing stemming back to an acute stress from working under an abusive boss. The revelations are often alarming. Mostly unexpected. The results are always beautiful. The unpredictability keeps me on my toes, especially with new people. But it also keeps my nerves up as I prepare myself for anything.

So while I'm already feeling my regular nerves, the topic of airplane travel adds a bit more discomfort for me. I flew a couple times as a child, but in college, thirty-five of my schoolmates were killed in a plane that was blown up by terrorists over Scotland in 1989. Without any post-trauma counseling, my brain wired itself to associate planes with terror. In other words, thinking of all the possible mishaps that can lead to my death in the sky, I never allowed myself to default to the comforting logic of, "It can't happen to me." Instead, I hear: *It can happen to me*, shouting through all reason.

When I saw the appointment note sent up to me by the general practice staff, mentioning a recommendation to help Vanessa address the stress of flying, I felt challenged. It weighed on me that I shared the same problem as she wanted to resolve. I took an extra few moments to prepare myself before I walked to the reception area.

Vanessa was sitting alone and waiting. Our reception area was busy. Near her were some of the general practice patients: moms with children, a man reading *The Economist,* another man in steel-toed work boots checking in for blood work.

Vanessa wasn't reading. She was sifting through her purse, pulled out a folded note, zipped her bag, and then noticed me. She slipped the note into her back pocket and stood to greet me with a smile and a handshake.

Our smiles deepened as she stood and noticed we were wearing matching turquoise blouses. I have never understood the phenomenon that happens when the same colors are inadvertently worn in a group at the same time. At schools, work, and even conferences, I've arrived wearing a muted teal blouse only to notice four other people sitting at my table selected the same obscure hue that morning. Lighthearted jokes about being "wardrobe psychics" would circulate. It's been a common occurrence that I have never taken the time to analyze. Vanessa's blouse was knitted silk with flecks of deep blue against the turquoise yarn. I wore a standard button down turquoise shirt with embroidered floral details on the collar. We both wore dark jeans that could pass as casual professional attire and the practical black Dansko clogs.

Inside the time of our quick handshake greeting, we exchanged a knowing chuckle without elaborating on the apparent wardrobe coincidence. But Justyna, the front desk manager, playfully suggested, "Did you two call each other when you got dressed today?" Vanessa and I ascended the stairs as we escaped the friendly banter in the waiting room.

In my office, I invited Vanessa to sit to review her intake form. There was nothing out of the ordinary until I saw her comment next to "Reason for Visit." She wrote, "Freaking out about my flight to Japan." I laughed out loud.

I looked up. "Well, that's honest."

"Yup," she smiled back.

"I'm no expert in flying without anxiety—we're going to rely on your energy body's wisdom."

As I began my hands-on work, Vanessa's energy felt like plastic Saran Wrap around her skin. I sensed, predictably, a deep fear.

Within several concentrated minutes with my hands practically pulling off the plastic wrap, her life force easily transmuted to a balanced, flexible body ready to support her full health. From here, I followed her intention to release the anxiety of flying.

Suddenly, I was pulled toward her fifth-chakra area as if a gentle magnet directed me toward her neck and jaw. I know this to be the area of open communication in the practice of clear listening and speaking. The color associated with this energy area is blue with variations from cobalt to pale sky. Color, in this case, is an impression. Whenever I am asked about the significance of a chakra color, I explain that color is a language beyond words that holds a meaningful vibration on the light spectrum.

With deep blue as my only focus, I stayed near her fifth chakra at her collarbone, which is the area connected to her heart chakra. The heart chakra is also known as the fourth chakra. This is the green chakra that holds love, grief, and the desire to live wholeheartedly.

Translating this colorful swirl of blue and green that was part of her own body's healing mechanisms, I was filled with a spectrum of emotions but no words.

In the quantum physics discussion around human healing, there is an idea that we can energetically travel beyond the limitations of time, space, and distance. I have found, in some cases, that I can "travel" to the origin of a wound. It is less about science fiction movie plots like *Back to the Future*, and more about unfolding the power of memory. Memory has a dynamic energy that seems to want to participate in offering insight to relieve pain and restore health. Harnessed this way, memory is a healing force like no other.

With Vanessa, I carried my hand through an imaginary time line to give context to quantum energy. I went back ten years, then twenty years, and eventually back thirty-three years. Thirty-three years ago a significant event informed her belief in flight and travel. Unexpectedly, I was met with an impression of elation, and a sense of overwhelming joy as if she absolutely loved to fly. We worked in silence as I lightly cleared any blocks alienating her scared self from the ecstatic child who flies happily.

With my hands still on her quantum time line, I suddenly felt a sharp drop away from joyful well-being to disorientation. I was in that thirty-three-year-ago time frame.

Vanessa's breath pattern shifted—a deep inhale with a slow jagged exhale, and I knew we had found a crucial block.

"Vanessa, do you recall a significant life event that may have once led you to love flying, but then it became scary?" I asked.

She just kept silent.

"Maybe you were too young," I suggested.

"No," Vanessa spoke but didn't open her eyes. "My first flight was hellish. I was nine years old."

I craned my next back to her paperwork. Her birthdate showed she was born in 1969. It was exactly thirty-three years ago.

"This is important for you. Tell me more about your first flight."

Vanessa went on to describe that trip with her elderly, blind godfather to the Midwest. She was assigned to be his travel companion, "sort of like a seeing-eye child instead of a seeing-eye dog," she explained. He had only lost his sight in the last four years of his life, but he confided to young Vanessa that he would be seeing her again soon. He told her his blindness was a temporary condition. Her nine-year-old self believed that, too.

She told me she remembered looking out the plane's window and describing the cotton-ball-like clouds and farmland like checkerboards. In his blindness, her godfather could explain engine sounds and the flight's elevation based on her descriptions of the view. They were bonding on this adventure across America, her sight and his life experience complementing each other's journey.

Like so many travel stories, there was a plot twist at the halfway point. In

Vanessa's story, it was a storm that caused an unplanned layover at the Denver airport.

She mentioned this detail and returned to silence for a few moments. Suddenly her breath became shallow and quick as she remembered something.

"After two or three hours of waiting, my godfather began to lose his grip on reality." Vanessa began to cry. "He began hallucinating and believed he was imprisoned. He was banging his cane on the airport floor demanding release."

I handed her a tissue while she continued, "Then a flight attendant walked over and, like a strict schoolteacher, told him to behave. I remember the firm warning from that woman in uniform—she threatened to remove him from the passenger list. He wouldn't be allowed to fly."

As if I was a static electricity conductor, at that moment I felt a shock from Vanessa's heart to my hands. Her chin quivered as she remembered begging her elderly godfather, her only travel companion, to stop yelling and stop banging his cane on the floor. But the more she pleaded through her tears, she recalled, the louder he protested.

"I demand to know what's going on. Why am I here, why am I here?" she repeated his shouts from thirty-three years ago.

In my office, Vanessa then became very quiet for three, four, five long minutes. She was distant and calm.

"That was your very first flight?" I interrupted the silence.

"As far as I know it was. I had never seen the clouds as cotton balls before that," she said.

"Did you eventually get safely to your destination?" I asked.

"I guess so, but I have no idea how it worked out. I don't really rememb..." she stopped abruptly.

Just then her field shifted under my hands, as if a cloak pulled away to unveil an even quieter body. Now a gentle magnetic force hovered near her head. I followed a lavender sixth-chakra energy to the field above her forehead. But there wasn't a sensation, only nothingness. I continued in silence for a whole forty-five minutes. I'd never experienced such a vacancy of a life force. The air around her body was just . . . air. I simply observed. It was unusual. I embraced it.

After this long wait, I phrased the question differently. "Do you recall how you reached your destination?"

No words, but her fingers twitched to indicate she needed more time before speaking.

In silence, I returned to her heart energy that I can only describe as exuding an intelligent and boundless love.

The session time was over. "Good work today," I assured her. "How do you feel?"

"I feel more relaxed. Can I schedule again before the trip?" she asked from the table.

"Take a couple of minutes to integrate. I'll leave you alone in the room to collect yourself and connect with your awareness of this early memory. We can book you when I come back. You seemed to go to a deep place . . ."

Five minutes passed and I gently knocked on the door. Vanessa was sitting up holding her face in her hands.

"I know I need to go, but I can't get off this table yet, I'm sorry," she whispered.

Something profound had returned to Vanessa—her field was fortified again. I told her she did not need to rush this moment. I leave plenty of time between my scheduled clients.

"What happened?" I wondered out loud to her. "You seem upset but energetically stronger at the same time."

"I am. When you walked away, I remembered the rest of the trip. It was a miracle. How could I have forgotten?" Vanessa asked herself, then continued, "As I attempted to calm my godfather, I put an arm around him and spoke through my tears to please stop yelling, we are going to get in trouble, please stop, I kept asking. I was beginning to beg."

"Then," she paused to catch her breath, "you know how some airport seats are back to back in the waiting area?"

"Sure, yes," I said.

"A couple, a woman and a man, traveling together, turned around and mercifully interrupted us. The woman apologized for intruding but said she thought she could help. Out of childhood instinct, I didn't trust them at first. Another airline attendant noticed the interaction—probably because the cane stopped banging—and also stood with us.

"While a rainstorm grounded planes and washed down the Rocky Mountains, a married couple from Boston explained that they were traveling from the School for the Blind in Watertown, Massachusetts and if the airline could arrange it, they would change seats to escort us the rest of the way to Wyoming until my godfather and I would be met by family at the arrival gate . . .

"That's how I got to my destination," she declared with an easy smile. "I wonder if they were actually real people or angels. It was the closest thing I've ever experienced to angels appearing. And maybe they were just a regular couple sitting in the right place at the right time."

"What do you think?" I asked.

"Both," she unzipped her purse to grab her calendar.

We laughed at the simplicity of this breakthrough.

"Can you remind me of all this at our next session before I leave for Japan?"

"Sure, just tell me what to say in my notes here—it's your miracle after all."

"Write this down: There is boundless love inside of life's adventures," she said. "I can't wait to go to Japan."

"Yes," I looked at the clock and handed her my notes. "How about you call me when you get back from Japan?" I suggested.

We both smiled, knowing a big healing shift was complete.

I woke up as our plane began its descent into Florida and I noticed my sweaty palms were cooling on my heart. I looked over and saw my son still leaning into the window to peer at the clouds below. I smiled knowing I was feeling calmer. He looked over at me again, "Take my seat, Mom, and you look out the window, too. Do you want to, Mom?"

"No thanks, buddy," I kept smiling, "I'm comfortable right where I am."

THE GOOD MEDICINE
OF EVERYDAY MIRACLES

Medicine Bottle #31

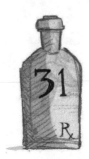

DENVER ANGELS

Angels can be people, too. No kidding. And people can be angels, too.

Think about it. You have been in the presence of people who work like angels. Qualities can be: a selfless character, a caring attitude, an unexpected resourcefulness, kindness beyond measure, bravery on purpose, and a lifestyle of connecting with others.

Open your heart to memories of times you were helped in miraculous ways. Try to remember how you were helped.

Can you list a few examples from your life when you may have witnessed an everyday miracle?

1. _____

2. _____

3. _____

This is your prescription for the Good Medicine of Everyday Miracles.

May experience an increased ability to detect the protective
and healing forces around you.

chapter 32

HAWK

I notice birds above me when I'm driving. I observe birds flying in formation or perched on a wire. I think they bring me comfort—something about the way these free creatures can fly while I am glued to the earth by gravity.

Some birds have beautiful markings. Early that morning, a cobalt-blue bird with a tangerine chest landed on a limb outside my kitchen window. Its beauty entranced me away from the tedious indoor task of dishes. It looked like a cartoon drawing of a red bellied robin, but a little smaller and a lot more colorful. So after a long day at the office with several back-to-back sessions and a meeting, it was no wonder I kept watching the sky for signs of birds.

My commute is part of my job. While I'm driving, I slow down my thoughts and consider the day's upcoming clients. There's one special part of the road where seagrass waves twelve months a year and the highway begins to split toward Maine. That's usually where I start to prepare.

This is the everyday sacredness where I change my focus to a more spiritual place while still cruising at sixty miles per hour.

In this same place, on the commute home away from my clients, I begin to "bless and release" all the happenings of the workday. And I begin to think about my life at home again: meals, laundry, homework, and bills.

On this particular day, green growth was pushing through the dry winter brown. Suddenly, I noticed a gull-sized bird bouncing sunlight off its feathers and I wondered how strange it was to see a gull this far inland. It's only a couple of miles to the salt water, but I have never noticed a gull near this part of the highway. It was converging with my path, swooping downward toward my car.

Suddenly, it stopped flying and fell straight to the ground. I was confused and concerned as the only witness to this harsh ending. Still driving, I turned my head to see that it wasn't white or gray but rather milky amber with white flecks. It was a hawk on the ground with big bent wings, all symmetry gone.

I slowed my car. My small rearview mirrors showed me nothing other than the blurred guardrails. It was Passover evening and the next day was Easter day—a weekend full of holidays. I wanted to get home, but I was compelled to check up on the well-being of this hawk. I exited turning right, and right, and then right again. Driving toward the same spot on the ramp where I saw the incident, I pulled over and googled the number for the Center for Wildlife in Maine.

"Wildlife Center," a young woman's voice answered. "This is Lindsey."

"Hi, I'm glad you're there." I was genuinely surprised when a real person answered. "I'm calling from route ninety-five, and I just saw a hawk fall from the sky. I'm going back to rescue it, or at least get the body in case it's a bird flu case or something like that. It was so bizarre to just witness a bird fall out of the sky."

"Okay, ahh, good . . . well . . . if it's still alive you will need to bring the bird up here, but, well, a hawk can be really kind of dangerous with a sharp beak and claws that rip . . . You don't want an angry hawk in your car. Do you have a towel and a large box?" I can hear loud chatter in her background. "Our falcon is telling me what she thinks of hawks."

"Well no, not a box," I was pretty certain this bird did not survive. "But I have a big shopping bag from Marshall's and a load of sheets." I started to drive again to circle back to the same spot.

Lindsey warned, "That bag won't work if the hawk comes back to life in your car. You need a real box."

"Hold on, I'm getting closer to the area I last saw . . . and I'm slowing down . . . I'm going to check for blood and see if it's moving at all."

"Well, be careful if you pull over . . ."

"I will, I promise . . . it's just that . . ." I was driving too slow for the speed limit on the ramp, so I shifted my focus back and forth from searching the ground to watching for any upcoming cars behind me. "I just can't find the exact place. I don't see the bird . . . it's not here anymore. Weird . . . where is it?" I spoke my thoughts out loud to the Wildlife Center. "It was right in the open, and now it's nowhere to be found."

"Oh," her voice smiled, "that hawk was hunting. They fly straight down and land with wings out for protection and balance. It could look like a fall from the sky to you."

Huh. So that hawk flew away with a fresh kill at the very same time I imagined an elaborate tragedy and rescue.

"Thank you so much, Lindsey" I apologized." You must think I'm a nut."

"No, we appreciate you trying to help the birds, and now you know that we're here seven days a week."

"Well, thanks so much and really, I'll let you go. Bye!"

"Call anytime. Bye!"

If only I steered toward the highway and ignored my suspicions about this mysterious bird dropping out of the sky, I would have already been home with my family.

But I earned a fresh look at my utter separation from nature's constant cycle. If I didn't know better, I'd have claimed a resurrection . . .

BEFORE

It happened before our species wrapped our auric field in shoes and bras and neckties. In the times before we blocked out our natural sensors with floors and ceilings. Before stories were scripted, and even before sounds were shaped into letters. There was a long time when the plants, animals, weather, and the vast sky was the alphabet for our only language.

Nothing has changed, and yet everything has changed now. The ancient language of the natural world is instilled in everyone. We can resuscitate it back from the edge of our collective memory and imagine a story for the tribe.

ॐ

On my bookshelf next to my bed, Jamie Sams and David Carson's book *Medicine Cards* had a ragged purple cover that's stained and faded with red magic marker scribbles on the back. But the pages remain clean and unripped. This book is a written apothecary where each short chapter connects the reader to a Native North American animal translation of old healing meanings. Wolf, Owl, Squirrel, Bear, Lynx, Armadillo, and forty-six more species are described for their medicinal messages. If an animal appears unusually on a walk, on a drive, in your path, and even in a dream, pay attention because the natural world is telling you something you need to know.

Sams and Carson translate the oldest language: "*When you call upon the power of an animal, you are asking to be drawn into complete harmony with the strength of that creature's essence. Gaining understanding from these brothers and sisters of the animal kingdom is a healing process, and must be approached with humility and intuitiveness.*"

Hawk is the second power animal featured in their book. Eagle is first. Eagle holds the energy of the Spirit. Hawk is the Messenger.

A hawk fell from the sky at the exact same moment I passed by. I played the fool, imagining that I witnessed a mysterious demise of this tremendous red-tailed bird. As I plotted my rescue and circled back on the limited path of the paved road, the broad wings carried this bird-of-prey back to his perch to savor its fresh small catch.

As I drove the rest of the way home that evening, I was left to wonder what I'd learned from this hawk's message.

THE GOOD MEDICINE OF SPIRIT ANIMALS

Medicine Bottle #32

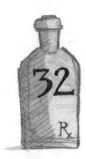

HAWK

Just like the chapter "Signs" describing the words that had nothing to do with *my* life, I saw a hawk fall out of the sky and I assumed "death."

The hawk was not a victim and the hawk was not even sick. I was the one who got it wrong.

Is there a perceived problem that you are mis-reading? What if it's not even a problem at all?

Identify one "problem" that you are struggling with:

_____

Look at it clearly from the sharp and high perspective of Hawk as a power spirit animal. Hawks' eyes can see both colors and heat that's undetectable to humans.

Hawk is the Messenger. Close your eyes. Ask for a message as you imagine your "problem" flying away before you can circle back to the scene.

This is your prescription for the Good Medicine of Spirit Animals.

May begin to see the whole picture and realize it's better
than you thought, not worse.

chapter 33

WHAT HOLDS US TOGETHER

O n the day before Maggie's service, I needed to deliver photographs to Reverend Scrogin's widow, Sue Ellen, who lived up the hill from the church.

Worcester, Massachusetts is a city with seven hills. Driving past the art museum and the university there is a beautiful brick church with a grand steeple on the corner of Salisbury Street. It sits at the bottom of one of the hills. The land for this church was donated by the neighbors, who had a luxurious Tudor estate with walls landscaped by grape vines twining through their property. As these homeowners were members of the church congregation, they generously donated the land. However, as real estate abutters, they withheld the tradition of a church bell in the sales agreement. They never wanted to be disturbed or awoken by loud gonging right outside their window.

I know this story because this is the legend of why we don't have a bell. I grew up in this church community. This was the place I first understood religion. From preschool to college, I was raised here.

When I was ten years old, our minister stood in front of the congregation and with tears in his eyes confessed that his marriage was ending in divorce. This was the 1970s. The church was not prepared to keep a divorced man as a leader. After a tumultuous debate among congregants, his resignation was accepted. He was replaced by a former college football player who was an NFL prospect with a soft southern accent. The new minister was Reverend Michael Scrogin.

Even as a child, I loved the way Reverend Scrogin's sermons folded quotes from current literature and personal anecdotes into the Sunday morning message. His lessons were both gentle and bold. Most memorable was a sermon titled, "Thinking The Unthinkable" where he called upon us in the marble sanctuary to invest in peace and support nuclear disarmament efforts. Yet another sermon was titled "Sometimes You Just Have to Try" as he shared the biblical message of doing what's best and trying your best even when the outcome isn't guaranteed. He illuminated this point by telling a story about his daughter, Sarah, who on a Wednesday night had worked up the confidence with a friend to ask for a midweek sixth-grade slumber party. Although he explained in the sermon that his parental answer was always going to be a "no" on a weeknight, he highlighted the tenacity of his daughter and her friend for the courage to simply try. There is spiritual value in "just trying" he said that day. Trying is a form of hope. And hope is sacred to living fully bound with love, he taught us that Sunday.

Reverend Mike Scrogin could craft a sermon. Often, in my early twenties, I would return to this church alone to listen to his brilliant weavings. And he was gifted with understated humor that provided a reliable laughter that would rumble out from even the most stoic members of the church. More than his words, I felt safer around Reverend Scrogin than anyplace else in the world. I'm not sure that I believed in God, but I believed in Michael Scrogin.

When I was twenty-five years old, he died after a short battle with stomach cancer. He was fifty-one. Devastation doesn't begin to describe my reaction. His memorial service was two full hours. I wept in the corner of a pew the whole time.

❧

Seven years later, his wife, Sue Ellen, hired my husband to photograph Sarah's wedding. Brian agreed to do the photography under the condition that he wouldn't charge for it. My husband knew that this family, the Scrogins, had an infinitely special place in my heart.

The night of the wedding, after the cake was cut and the groom drove the bride away, Sue Ellen handed me a thank-you note that I tucked in my pocket to read later. Once we loaded the equipment into our vehicle, we sat in a parking lot eating leftovers. I remembered I had the note. As I unfolded it, out dropped a check for twelve hundred dollars with an earnest request to accept her payment. This was more money than my husband would have ever charged. This was a pot of gold for our lives as working artists.

Hoping that she would like the wedding photos, I arranged to drop them off personally on my way to Maggie's house that morning. I sat at Sue Ellen's kitchen table sifting through the wedding pictures, which naturally became an inspiration to chat about memories.

I told Sue Ellen how I wished I could ask her husband for his advice to lead Maggie's service. I asked her about Reverend Scrogin's insights and his approach to crafting a meaningful and poignant memorial service.

"Well," she started, "he would take lots of time to talk to the family. And talk to close friends, too—as much as possible—to get their stories. And, actually . . ." she interrupted her own thought. "Do you know the story of Mike's last words?" she asked me, almost rhetorically.

"No," I said. My heartbeat sped up. I'd never heard it. *How could I have?* I wondered.

Sue Ellen continued, "Well, he had become very weak, and he asked me to grab a pen and paper to write something down to tell the kids. He had said so little in the last days, I was frantic to find something to write with. I expected he had a lost insurance number or some bookkeeping detail to share. So I sat ready to write down a set of numbers. But instead, he described something else. He told me, 'They're placing stones around my body to act as passageways to openings. There is so much more that holds me together than just skin. This has been a huge disruption in my life,'" Sue Ellen paused.

I caught my breath.

There is so much more that holds us together than just skin, I thought.

Hearing this, my worlds folded, and reality became just wavelengths. I couldn't speak, but I'm sure as my throat closed, my jaw dropped open. Just days before, without any instruction, I placed stones around Maggie's body by instinct alone. I would have never been in the room with Maggie's body if not for the broken van, Rudy the corpse mover, the construction workers on coffee break, Beth's courage, and Sage's patience with it all.

This has been a huge disruption in my life. Again, I could not process these very last words in their whole form. Was he speaking from the other side of his life already? The cancer was taking his body away. But in his last words he had gone from preacher to an on-the-scene notetaker. Who are "they"? Who are the ones placing stones around his body? The man had a reverence for words, and he gathered his strength to speak these last sentences. The word choice of *disruption* was his way of sharing his experience.

I told Sue Ellen about the stones I placed around Maggie's body, but she was still reminiscing, "I remember feeling angry writing the word 'disruption,' which felt like the most ridiculous understatement to what I was experiencing. But I'm glad I wrote it down because those were some of his last words."

I'm glad she wrote it down, too.

After a long hug, I left the large stack of wedding photos at the kitchen table and continued my ride to Maggie's house.

Driving up Salisbury Hill, I passed my old neighborhood with the sidewalks I had walked to and from my elementary and middle schools for a decade. It is true what they say in each generation—I'd walk over a mile to get there, even in the snow and the rain. Through puddles and hot afternoons and snowbanks and icy slopes and crispy dry autumn leaves, those walks did me good.

My car would arrive too quickly at Maggie's house. I needed time to think and more time to prepare. Maggie had died only four days ago and my heart felt too heavy to lead this celebration.

I pulled over into the sandy parking lot next to Indian Lake.

"They're placing stones around my body that act as passageways."

His briefest sermon. Written down for his children.

"There is so much more than skin that holds me together."

What is it that holds *us* together? What part of him will travel through this passageway. Who was placing the stones?

"This has been a huge disruption in my life."

I imagined Reverend Scrogin's next sermon, if he had lived, with titles like "Death Is Just a Disruption," or "Disrupting Our Beliefs" or "When Cancer Disrupts Our Life." I wish I could have listened to any one of those imagined sermons, but as I looked out at the lake, I knew that the place of understanding the disruption was beyond words. It was even beyond reference. That moment of leaving his body was a disruption.

The lake water was choppy that morning. I watched a few ducks swim along the banks of the lake.

I would miss Maggie.

More than skin holds us together.

I thought I may know what these words meant; how more than our skin holds what is on the inside, our soul.

But what is our soul? Is it this energy that I'm discovering through my hands? I wondered about the energy that communicates through my heart—is that what holds us together?

In front of me, a flock of geese poured down onto the lake gliding across the water in their landing. Together. We are together, connected, even beyond our skin. In life and also in death.

Sue Ellen had answered my question by sharing these last words of a great preacher. *They're placing stones around my body to act as passageways to openings. There is so much more that holds me together than just skin. This has been a huge disruption in my life.*

I started my car and drove a short seven more miles to Maggie's house to prepare. The dogs barked at my arrival. Plans were solidified.

The next day I got there early. The music played. We cooked for the gathering. Guests began to arrive. More guests. More barking. More food. I spoke about love and loving Maggie. Others spoke about Maggie and more love, too. I shared the quote from Reverend Scrogin. Then I led a moment of silence. Until the dogs barked again. And for the rest of the evening the music played on as we celebrated Maggie's life.

THE GOOD MEDICINE OF LOVE
Medicine Bottle #33

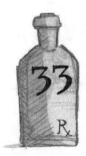

WHAT HOLDS US TOGETHER

Think about this; if you're fortunate enough, you'll have a chance to share your last words. You may even bear witness to the experience of leaving your body behind. Will you have something to say? Maya Angelo sent a final message through social media before she died: "Listen to yourself and in the quietude you may hear the voice of God," she wrote.

There is no reason to wait until your very last words. That time will come someday. This is your time to write a message to everyone who wants to hear about your life's wisdom. Write down what matters most. By doing this now, you may have even more wisdom when it is your final turn. Take your time.

Give yourself permission to write your "last words" on this page.

_____

_____

_____

_____

_____

_____

This is your prescription for the Good Medicine of Love.

May experience renewed life. Spontaneous creativity will occur.
Be prepared for a sudden onset of peace and healing.

chapter 34

BEANSTALK

Jared had cancer. He was in his early thirties. He reported that his recent courses in chemotherapy and radiation were measurably successful. He had just started an experimental therapy medicine at Massachusetts General Hospital in Boston. He had an advanced diagnosis. I had seen Jared for energy work every six weeks for over a year.

"I want to try something different today," Jared announced. He hadn't yet sat down.

"And I specialize in different," I joked.

"I've got some of this stuff under control, you know—my meds, my doses, my nutrition, your chakra stuff . . ." He scratched the back of his head as he looked at me. "But a big question keeps coming up."

"What's that?" I leaned forward as he sat down.

"God."

"God?"

"Yeah, when you hear those famous words 'you have cancer' you can't help feeling a little more curious about God. Do you get what I mean?" he asked.

"I'm listening . . ." I answered.

"I wonder about death, and I wonder about pain, and who gets hurt, and who gets to live."

I nodded wordlessly.

"I think about that giant in the clouds," he continued. "From that fairy-tale," he snapped his fingers. "What's that one called?"

"Jack in the Beanstalk," I recalled.

"Yes!" he pointed at me. "That giant with the golden eggs who eats little boys. The boys who climb to the clouds. How magic is a beanstalk that leads little kids to such danger? I don't like that story. And I'm starting to wonder if I got God mixed up with that giant."

In quiet recognition, I listened. A giant above the clouds being confused with an image of God? It sounded like a familiar mix-up to me, too.

"I want to focus on that today," he leaned back and looked out the room's only window.

As soon as we began the energy work, I felt a heaviness drain like a warm oil from his feet. Next, I hovered my hands over his abdominal area, where his cancer originated. A well of energy swirled there as I stayed for several minutes.

Then above his rib cage—where his heart chakra spins—about twelve inches above his body, I felt a magnetic sensation. His energy was expanding around his heart with great force. The whole room seemed to fill with a gentle expansion of the space. I was washed with a sense of big love. The feeling of joy, sorrow, grace, anticipation, and gratitude all twisted into a strand of love. I kept my hands in place above his heart.

"Can you feel that?" I found myself interrupted by my own voice.

"I feel a presence—something about my question," Jared answered with his eyes still closed.

"So do I."

"I get it," Jared rested his hands on his chest. "This feels nothing like the cruel giant, but it feels gigantic."

I waited for him to say more as I worked with his energy in silence.

"It's love everything. In capital letters," Jared said with the calmest exhilaration. "LOVE EVERYTHING."

I stayed with that thought. I felt it, too.

The very good.

The very bad.

The love of everything.

Are we free to just love all of life?

"I don't want to come back from here," he whispered.

"You're in no rush," I replied.

He started to cry silently with tears flowing over his temples. I dried the sides of his face with tissues and kept working with him for thirty more minutes. Then, I could feel a lightness in his abdominal area that wasn't there before.

When I left the room to make notes, it was like stepping into another climate. My colleagues were chatting, my cell phone lit up with text messages, and a car insurance payment reminder buzzed. I tried to hold on to the energy of my room, but I could only remember LOVE EVERYTHING, LOVE EVERYTHING. So that's all I wrote.

When I returned, Jared was waiting in the chair.

"I think we went somewhere today," I smiled.

"I think so, too," I could see his face beaming even as he looked down to tie his shoes.

"I don't think you'll need another appointment for a while," I admitted.

He looked up quickly, "I was thinking the same thing!"

"Good work, my friend," I smiled.

"Yeah, good work to you, too."

Three months later, an email arrived from Jared:

Hey, Hilary, I thought you'd be less than surprised to know that I'm officially cancer-free. I know I was helped along by great medicine and even better doctors. You kept me "healthy" even at my sickest moments. But mostly Hilary, I want to thank you for helping me with my BIG question. You wrote it down for me: LOVE EVERYTHING. It was the final prescription for my health. In our last session, I felt toxins leave my body as I replaced it all with love. Or I should say, LOVE. I think that's it. I'm grateful for your help getting me here.

Goodbye for now,
Jack (get it?)

I wrote back.
Dear "Jack,"

You're right. I'm not surprised. On so many levels, I'm not surprised at all. Thanks for the very good news.

Warmly,
Hilary

EPILOGUE

A year after my mother died, I decided to locate the fossil from nine-year-old Ella's birthday party. My mom had gone through the passageways to the cosmos. That fossil was my reminder that our wise souls are like prehistoric ferns pressed into earth. But I couldn't find any part of this fossil at my house. I searched for it feverishly and furiously, but the fossil was gone.

I recalled that the girls from the party had kept small pieces of the fossil, but I wondered if I had given away the big rock, too. About an hour later, I remembered. I had given the big fossil to Murphy.

❦

"Do you see this line splitting the two sides?" Murphy asked, showing me a stone larger than his hand that looked like a slice of a two-layer birthday cake. It was orange on one side with a stream of white in the middle, and gray on the other side. He explained, "This is my healing rock. It represents the before and the after."

"The before and after of what?" I was curious.

"The *before* I was sick and the *after* I'm healed."

He handed me the rock, which was heavier than I expected. "Is this granite from New Hampshire?" I pointed to the gray part of the stone.

"I carried it home from the mountain I lived on in Korea," Murphy said. "I was told the mountain was sacred. I was on opposite sleep schedules with the only other soldier there. We almost never saw each other, but we both decided to take a stone to remember that majestic mountain." With his hands free as I held his stone, Murphy took off his backpack and sat down. "As we activated and deactivated the nuclear warheads every day, we agreed our mountain must have been watching over us."

"This is taken from a sacred mountain?" I asked, examining the rock.

"It was sacred, but not in the way I thought it would be. The mountain wasn't overpowering. It was peaceful. In fact, the first real peace I ever knew. It was my home. I wasn't supposed to take any rocks from the mountain, but I needed a piece to carry with me. It's the before and it's the after."

I handed the stone back to Murphy. He only smiled.

"Keep it," he said.

"It belongs to you," I protested.

"It belongs to the mountain. Give it to someone who needs it. Someone else who comes to see you. See this line in the middle," he pointed to it again. "It's the change that comes to heal us. That line marks the moment of change. I don't need it anymore. I'm on the healing side now."

I sensed Murphy knew his disease had healed him. We had walked some of this journey together. At that moment, neither of us knew the full outcome of his cancer. It would be months before we had our cancer-free hug in the parking lot. Nevertheless, I held onto the stone.

"I have something for *you* then, my friend," I said and walked over to the shoebox stored safely in my bookshelf. "This is from Canada. It's some kind of slate, but see, there's a plant fossilized here."

Murphy took the rock with both hands.

"I like the fern, that's got to be old," he said.

I told him the story of Ella's birthday party and about Olivia, the girl who spoke with this fossil. "She told me this fossil knows about the beginning of us," I said. "Us humans."

"Kids know these things," Murphy said, as he flipped the rock over twice and then handed it back to me.

"No, you keep it," I said.

"I think you need it here," he argued.

"It's been here for a long time," I said. "Bring it home, even just to put it in your garden."

"I will," Murphy said with sudden grace in his acceptance.

"Do you think this fossil is connected to the soul of the original fern?" I wondered out loud.

"I think the fern was perennial and grew stronger year after year," he answered. "Wherever this stone came from, I bet if we go back to that place, there's a fern still growing there today."

"A geologist told me that this rock is over 150 million years old." I giggled at the immenseness of that number.

"Yep," Murphy didn't flinch.

"But I bet you're right, there's a fern still growing in that exact spot where it was found," I agreed.

"No doubt about it," he said as he packed the fossil into the side pocket of his backpack.

I placed Murphy's rock from the Korean mountain on the small wooden table between us. Then, as we settled in to begin our weekly session, I asked, "What should we work on today?"

ACKNOWLEDGMENTS

If I could climb to the top of a mountain and shout out my sincere devotion for every client, I would still be up on the summit outpouring my appreciation. But my oath of confidentiality is too strong and too sacred to whisper a word. You will each need to know who you are when I say how profoundly grateful I am to be part of your healing journey. I am a student of your healing body's wisdom. I am grateful for every moment we've had together. I wrote this book in honor of all I've learned so far.

Thank you, Mom—I hope you get to read this somewhere in the nearby cosmos. And thank you, Dad. I know you'll get to read this, and that gives me more joy than you can imagine. I thank my grandparents who haunt me with happiness and a sense of belonging that still fills my heart. And I thank my godparents for watching over me from near and far.

Amanda Wood taught me that lists can be literature, too. Amanda is an exquisite writer. Her book of poems sits on my bedside as a touchstone to inspire me. Amanda leads the writing group where I belong at the Gloucester Writing Center. Thank you to all the women writers in our group. I'm going to trust in the power of the list.

I begin with Jessica Purdy, my poet-neighbor-teacher friend. I won the jackpot when we moved in across the street from Jess and her family. She taught me to unleash my analytical prose into the language of story.

I want to ask Jess, "How do I possibly write an acknowledgments page when my heart is so full for you and everybody who came before and after you?"

Marc Clopton can only be truly thanked with a deep bow to Bonnie-Jean Wilbur and Paul Wann. All three graced me with wisdom about the power of authentic expression. And then there is the absolute gift of Pearl herself. I hope Pearl gets to read this, too.

With this list, I'll start from the top, as I imagine Pearl wants me to. I can hear her toes tapping as she sings, "and a five, six, and a five, six, seven, eight . . . this time from the top."

Miriam Wolf taught me to work hard, be true, stay focused, and believe the human body is always communicating on behalf of its own health. She helped me heal. She helped me heal others. Miriam is a force for good health in this world.

Lisa Rudley and I met in Putney, Vermont, as Miriam's students. I'm glad I said yes to Ms. Rudley when she invited me to the Upper East Side to connect with the healing masters, Conor, Deborah, Jean, Susan, and Kim.

Dagny St. John, I also met you in Miriam's classroom, and yet I'm sure our friendship goes back lifetimes. May it go forward lifetimes, too.

To all my cousins, I know energy can not be created nor destroyed. But joy feels like new energy. That matters with us.

The McCann-McNally-Benson clan . . . may we all circle each other for generations forward.

My cousin Jill Keil is my anchor, my home away from home, my teacher through life, my great friend, and my family. I am who I am because she has always stood by me. You and Nick welcomed me over and over into your Vermont sanctuary and that has changed the trajectory of my entire life. Meghan, Galen, Silas, Joah, Hunter, Ellen, Malcom, Adam, Jolly, and Bobo, I love being part of your family.

I love and thank my family of origin of Mom, Dad, Judith, Hunter, and Caleb. And their beautiful families with Peter, Betsy, and Rachel. And my arms stretch around with love for your children: Tommy, Ella, Sadie, Coco, and Phoebe.

And deep gratitude to all of my extended family. We are a big, loving group of hunters and jewels gathering together.

I'm blessed by my family through my marriage, too. Mrs. Cathleen Crowley, Jim, Connie, John, Kev, Katie, Ed, Lee, Cathleen, Greg, Henry, Laura, Deb, Kitty, Jess, and Elaine. And further blessed by more fun-loving nieces and nephews: Jimson, Fallon, Athena, Sammy, Rachel, Conor, Shamus, Julia, Hannah, Cavan, Matty, Annah, Ella D., and Anna D.

All of this life orbits around the bright light of my absolute three: my husband, Brian, and my two boys that call me mom. Wyeth. William. How my boys arrived into this world five months apart is a story for another book. I say to you here, I'm so glad you did arrive. You are my middle, my beginning, and my ending. How we roll through life together is what truly matters most.

I again thank my mother for showing me the power of friendship. Her friends were her gold. To my dear friends, you've shaped these stories in more ways than I could ever count. You also know who you are in these mentions. You are my gold.

My professional family lives at Whole Life Health Care. I thank Amy Coombs, the founder, the guide, the caring practitioner, and the visionary of this extraordinary concept. I appreciate your wholehearted welcome to this warm center of integrative medicine. And for Elisabeth, I was lucky enough to find her long before I knew we'd be colleagues. Through these years, I'm grateful to integrate with superb holistic practitioners inside this big historical home for health care: Peggy, Melissa, Lisa G, Ranan, Rachel, Christina, Gi, Oz, Ryan, Kursten, Jennifer, Jessica, Carli, Ellen, Naomi, Kay, Catherine, Margaux, Julie, Tammy, and Dawn. And thanks to the incredible staff that runs the general family practice with a daily humanity that's both rare and wonderful in this world. Thanks to Bob, of course, who keeps the "Whole" in Whole Life Health Care. Cheryl, I thank you for inviting me on that snowy day. And I must ask, "Justyna, do you still remember snowy days?"

I'm grateful for my lifelong book club buddies in Exeter. As we keep reading for fun over tea and cocktails, may we always appreciate the power of books together.

For all my neighbors between Winter and Summer Street, thank you for growing up with me in the middle of my life. And with the prospect of another great neighborhood, I understand that writing in peace has everything to do with living in a kind community.

Jane Bernstein is my personal editor and the life coach who kept me on course. She has been my rock in many storms, and fair winds in many sails.

Lisa Tener brought my book to life and connected me with Jane. Engulfed in the sparkling morning light of the churning ocean, Lisa's classroom is an enchanted place to grow words into chapters.

Tatiana and I met at the best place and at the right time. I want to thank Tatiana in advance for all we will discover and for how far we will reach.

Kim Mack Rosenberg, for your keen eye, lioness heart, and connecting me to the great people of Skyhorse Publishing, I thank you with the loudest roar.

Thank you Tony Lyons, for believing in my manuscript and introducing me to Abigail Gehring.

Abigail, you've been a delight from our first introduction. Thanks for your savvy sensibility. Your calm and kind approach to creating literature is everything I could ever want from an editor for *The Power of Energy Medicine*. You've surrounded me with good energy in the very best way.

Dan Chartand, your bookstore flows with the love of literature, reading, and elevating authors. While I'm proud to join the rank of local author, I'm deeply appreciative for your role to get me here.

John Klossner, I've witnessed how stories unfold the moment your pencil touches your sketch pad. I'm honored to have your artwork touch these pages, too.

Lauren Walker, you put the magi back in magic. We reunited without any frenzied forces of social media. You were so gracious to read my book, and yet I could have never predicted that you'd love it. You helped me believe in this book. Let's keep weaving stories together.

Beth M., so filled with gratitude for the walks, the work, and your careful reading of my manuscript. You let me know I was on track and, therefore, I kept going. Your insider tip on how to be an A+ student arrived late in my life but, turns out, just in time.

Sally R., what is it like to be a great poet, a veteran nurse, and a seasoned gardener all in one place? You're a keeper of healthy souls. Thank you for welcoming me to walk on your path and sit under your tree.

Alethea Black, for bringing me into your world of great writing—I adore your gift with words and I'm honored that you adore mine.

Lisa Rockenmacher, as an early reader you encouraged me to write down the inside whispers that also belonged in these pages. I'm so grateful that I listened to you.

Beth W, you've been with me at two big deadlines—and you carried me bravely both times. Thanks for your fire. It matters.

My heart breaks open missing Ricardo and missing James—once connected, always connected.

Trisha, thank you for the laughs, and the trail runs, and for sharing Alexis. Let's always keep in touch.

There is so much more than skin that holds me together. Thank you Sue Ellen for sharing this message from Mike. Thank you, Joel and Sarah. Your dad's last words have become this whole book.

NOTES

NOTES

NOTES

NOTES

....
....
....
....
....
....
....
....
....
....
....
....
....
....
....
....
....
....

NOTES

NOTES

NOTES

NOTES

....

....

....

....

....

....

....

....

....

....

....

....

....

....

....

....

....

....

....

NOTES

....
....
....
....
....
....
....
....
....
....
....
....
....
....
....
....
....
....

NOTES

NOTES

....
....
....
....
....
....
....
....
....
....
....
....
....
....
....
....
....
....
....

NOTES

NOTES

NOTES

NOTES

NOTES